P9-EDV-609

ALSO BY KAREN R. KOENIG

The Rules of "Normal" Eating

The Food and Feelings Workbook

*What Every Therapist Needs to Know About Treating
Eating and Weight Issues*

Nice Girls
Finish Fat

PUT YOURSELF FIRST AND
CHANGE YOUR EATING FOREVER

KAREN R. KOENIG
LCSW, M.ED.

A FIRESIDE BOOK
Published by Simon & Schuster
New York London Toronto Sydney

Fireside
A Division of Simon & Schuster, Inc.
1230 Avenue of the Americas
New York, NY 10020

Some individuals in this book are composites.

Copyright © 2009 by Karen R. Koenig

All rights reserved, including the right to reproduce this book or portions thereof in any form whatsoever. For information address Fireside Subsidiary Rights Department, 1230 Avenue of the Americas, New York, NY 10020.

First Fireside trade paperback edition June 2009

FIRESIDE and colophon are registered trademarks of Simon & Schuster, Inc.

For information about special discounts for bulk purchases, please contact Simon & Schuster Special Sales at 1-800-456-6798 or business@simonandschuster.com.

The Simon & Schuster Speakers Bureau can bring authors to your live event. For more information or to book an event contact the Simon & Schuster Speakers Bureau at 866-248-3049 or visit our website at www.simonspeakers.com.

Designed by Jessica Shatan Heslin/Studio Shatan, Inc.

Manufactured in the United States of America

10 9 8 7 6 5 4 3 2

Library of Congress Cataloging-in-Publication Data
Koenig, Karen R., 1947–
Nice girls finish fat : put yourself first and change your eating forever / Karen Koenig.
p. cm.
"A Fireside Book."
1. Weight loss—Psychological aspects. 2. Reducing diets—Psychological aspects. 3. Health behavior. I. Title.
RM222.2.K5755 2009
613.2'5—dc22
                                                                      2009002278
ISBN-13: 978-1-4165-9264-8
ISBN-10:   1-4165-9264-4

This book is dedicated to
Lynda Pasqua,
without a doubt one of the nicest "girls"
anyone would ever want to know.

Acknowledgments

I am unbelievably fortunate to spend much of my time engaged in two activities I adore—treating clients in psychotherapy and writing. Therefore, my first burst of gratitude goes to the hundreds of disregulated eaters I've met and worked with over the years. Whenever I've gone into a (hopefully unnoticed) funk and felt hopeless about therapy *really* working to overcome eating and weight problems, you've heartened me with your courage and ability to change and renewed my faith in the process. And, speaking of faith, the second tip of my hat goes to Janice M. Pieroni, my agent, who had faith in me long before I realized I was full of ideas and had enough talent to convert some of them into books. Did I mention her hard work, sense of humor, insight, editing skills, levelheadedness, and nurturing abilities?

Much appreciation goes to Michelle Howry, Senior Editor, Touchstone/Fireside, Simon & Schuster, whose enthusiasm, gentle suggestions, and keen editing eye morphed *Nice Girls Finish Fat* from a manuscript with potential into a polished, professional piece of work I can be proud of. As always, never-ending thanks goes to my husband for being the man he is.

Contents

Introduction:
Nice Girls—Read This

How Is Being Nice a Vice?

Weight loss is a marathon, not a sprint—and rare is the habitual overeater who goes on a diet, loses twenty or fifty pounds, and coasts slimly through the rest of her days. If staying trim were that easy, I'd be out of my psychotherapy job as fast as you could say Nutrishake. Instead of miraculous, overnight, permanent transformation, the stream of women I've treated for eating and weight problems over the past three decades had to struggle and settle for modest successes in improving their relationship with food and the bodies their aspiring spirits inhabit.

It isn't that they aren't motivated—they are!—or that they don't work hard in therapy—they do! Their drive to eat normally and lose weight has the focus of a laser. Their diet histories could fill libraries. They've read all the weight-loss books, sat through the twelve-step meetings, swallowed the magic pills, and had their stomachs surgically sectioned and stapled. Their stories are unique yet oddly universal. These women have been there and done that and are *still* searching for the Holy Grail that will grant them peace with the bleeping scale.

As I sit and listen to the play-by-play of their lives, one thing becomes clear. It's not just their dysfunctional childhoods, crummy genetic loading, depression, or anxieties that hold them back from reaching their eating and weight goals. Nor is it their stressful jobs, loopy families, parched lives, or lackluster spouses or partners. What keeps them fat and stuck in the cookie jar, unable to climb out and stay out, is that *they're too damned nice!*

They *love* being nice. I do an exercise in the first session of my Quit Fighting with Food workshop in which I ask participants (who are—big surprise—mostly women) to share one thing they like about themselves. And what do most of them say? They beam and tell me *they're nice*, of course. Though many are highly educated and skilled, world traveled, at the peak of impressive careers, or have raised children alone with few resources except their own broad shoulders . . . they continue to believe that their most striking asset is "being nice." Not that there's anything wrong with it, as they say on *Seinfeld*, but come on. It makes me want to cry and shake some sense into them at the same time.

The women I treat are so übernice that they'd not only insist on giving you the blouse off their backs, they'd launder and press it first, wait around for you to put it on, then button it up for you! These kinds of women swell the ranks of the helping professions—teachers, nurses, secretaries, librarians, and (yup) therapists—in part because they are ultranurturing, self-effacing, unselfish, generous, and caring to a fault. The problem is that often their size grows as big as their hearts.

Now, before readers who think I'm maligning either "nice" or "fat" start to pen me hate mail, let me clear up a few things. *There is nothing inherently wrong with being either fat or nice.* My goal here isn't character assessment and it certainly isn't character assassination. *Au contraire*, I've spent the last thirty years trying to help nice, overweight women stop obsessing about food, get healthy, love their bodies whatever they weigh, and move on with life. My point is that there just might be a correlation between being nice and getting (and staying) fat. The possibility and nature of that link are what this book is about.

Naturally, not every nice woman has eating or weight issues . . . and every fat female isn't sweet as honey. And, yes, there are nice men who are fat, thin, and in between, along with portly gents who are dear dumplings and others who are boorish brutes. Frankly, from the limited number of overweight men I've counseled (they don't come to therapy in droves, mind you), I'd say the too-nice label fits them like an extralarge glove. In fact, they're as doggone pleasant and other-centered as the women I treat, so the correlation between chubby and caring might not be a boy-girl thing after all.

However, for the purpose of this book, gender is what it's all about—the way women are brought up and expected to be nice and how that thrust of socialization straitjackets them in their options, cookie-cutters their personalities, and catapults them headfirst into the Häagen-Dazs. In this culture, even in this day and age, there is a humongous difference between how women and men are raised and treated (never mind the scientific variance of gender genetics), which makes women win the niceness contest hands down.

I know all about it. I was once an overly nice girl turned woman myself—an overweight one, at that. It's not that I'm no longer affable and kind or that I've given up being giving. I haven't. But I work extra hard at not striving to be nice for nice's sake, as if it's the brass ring or an Olympic medal, the one defining word that sums up my entire existence. I've incorporated a sprinkling of "not nice" into my personality and—wonder of wonders—I am still standing. As I've gotten older, I've developed this crazy notion I can be anything I want to be, and that includes a giver *and* taker, a person who elbows herself up to the front of the line when need be *and* invites folks to step ahead of her just because I feel like it, a woman who finds pleasing herself one of life's underrated delights, yet who is considered by most people as caring, nurturing, generous, and, yes, downright nice.

This book is for all you women who know you're too nice, who recognize somewhere deep inside that overdoing for others leaves nothing for you, who don't get why you can't stop eating when you're not hungry, who feel the need to apologize for any particle of your being that isn't wholesome and angelic, who take care of others with love and take care of yourself with food, who work too hard on being perfect, live to please others, think no and say yes, and have to make things right for everyone.

Every chapter in this book speaks to niceness that is unhealthy in its extreme and keeps you joined at the hip with food. Think of these pages as guiding you through an annotated tour of Niceville, including the pitfalls of perfectionism, the hazards of food as self-care, the downside of doing everything yourself, the perils of having your needle permanently stuck in the yes groove, the masochism of trying to be all things to all people all the time, and the dangers of letting yourself get so stressed out that you're killing yourself because you can't stop worshipping at the altar of nice. By the time you're done reading, you'll understand how being too good and giving at your own expense encourages you to camp out in front of your refrigerator and skyrockets your risk of remaining overweight, unhealthy, and underhappy.

Along the way, you'll learn the life skills and self-care strategies needed to create a happy, fulfilling, successful life and stop abusing food. *Life skills* are general abilities for negotiating the world effectively, your basic tools for maximizing your potential. *Self-care strategies* are exactly what they sound like, the behaviors and activities you must engage in to keep yourself in good shape—physically, mentally, and emotionally. Skills and strategies are all learnable with drive, practice, and patience. No matter how young or old you are, you can learn to make choices that are *always* in your best interest.

Chapters include a host of activities and advice to help you pack your bag and make tracks out of Niceville:

- *Grab Your Thinking Cap* exercises focus your attention on the psychological, interpersonal, and social aspects of your life you need to understand in order to make meaningful change.

- *Nice Girl Recovery Tips* give you a heads-up on how to undo years of overly nice behavior and transform dysfunctional beliefs and behaviors.

- *No More Nice Girl Manifestos* are practical dos and don'ts for every wannabe former nice girl.

- *Meet One of the Nice Girls* vignettes tell the stories of aspiring saints like you who are learning to toss away their halos and stop abusing food and their bodies.

Think of it: You'll soon be the envy of all your Goody Two-shoes friends—basking in the warmth of people who can't do enough for *you*, leaving work on the dot of five heading for a well-deserved workout, and dancing the night away instead of taking care of your sister's kids while she's out on the town. By the end of this book, you'll have the wisdom and tools to give yourself a surgically safe nice-ectomy, put food in its rightful place, and get on with creating the life you've always wanted and deserve.

Nice Girls
Finish Fat

ONE

Sugar and Spice and Everything . . . Fattening?

What's a "Nice" Girl?

Since you picked up this book (and read the introduction), you probably have an inkling of what being "nice" is all about . . . and how it can get us into trouble. In most cases, it's what our well-intentioned parents taught us to be, what our misguided mothers and other female relatives modeled for us, and how we were told men wanted us to act if we ever planned on dating and getting married. If you need a reminder, nice equals good, pleasing, agreeable, caring, kind, and thoughtful.

There's nothing inherently wrong with any of these traits individually or collectively. In fact, they're a pretty lofty group of attributes to aspire to—as far as they go. And therein lies the rub. If you were brought up to be intelligent, assertive, autonomous, creative, self-assured, candid, honest, secure, and successful—as well as nice—it's okay to give this book to someone who needs it more than you do. But many of us were encouraged to choose *only* the nice crayon when shading in our personalities. We didn't get much chance to try out the rest of the gloriously screaming colors in the box and, therefore, became boringly, unhealthy, monochromatically nice.

Exactly how nice is too nice?

For the purpose of this book, let's say there's a difference between being *nice* and *too nice*, a workout that is so off the charts that it actually gives nice a bad name. So that we're all on the same page here, let's assume it's okay to be a sweetheart and an earth mother as long as you have the ability to turn off these traits and bring in the big guns of selfish, practical, confident, bold, bullish, driven, and outspoken when you need 'em. As the oracles advise, we need to be in balance.

How do you know if you're overdoing it with sweetness and light and jeopardizing your physical and emotional well-being? How do you make sure you're not so accustomed to being a dear and a darling that you fail to notice how sadly one-dimensional you've become? How do you push aside your fears about seeing yourself as you *really* are long enough to discover if you've got a halo welded to your head?

Here's how. Gulp a deep breath, aim for honest, take this little test, and find out what it has to say about your niceness level. (And please don't agonize over your answers. There are only twenty questions and they're all simple, declarative sentences. Hint: Not wanting to fail or make mistakes may be a big part of your problem.)

HOW NICE ARE YOU?

Write the number that best describes in general how you think, feel, or act:

1 = Rarely/Never   2 = Sometimes   3 = Often   4 = Always

_4_ 1. I jump in and take care of family members when others could but don't or won't.

_3_ 2. I feel guilty whenever I say no to family members or disappoint them.

_3_ 3. I avoid burdening family members with my problems.

_3_ 4. I put family members' needs before mine at my own expense.

_2_ 5. I take care of friends more than they take care of me.

_3_ 6. I feel guilty and bad whenever I say no to friends or disappoint them.

_2_ 7. I am there for friends even when they're not there for me.

_1_ 8. I put friends' needs before mine at my own expense.

_3_ 9. Even though it stresses me out, I push myself to give my all at work.

_____ 10. I pick up coworkers'/bosses' slack and rarely get credit for it.

_____ 11. People at work take advantage of my good and giving nature.

_____ 12. I stress myself out by saying yes to people when I know I should say no.

_____ 13. I feel in the wrong and apologize automatically even when I'm not at fault.

_____ 14. I keep silent about what's on my mind rather than speak up.

_____ 15. I feel that whatever I do isn't enough with friends, family, at work, and at play.

_____ 16. If I don't do something perfectly, I feel like a failure.

_____ 17. I'm mortified about making mistakes because of what people will think of me.

_____ 18. I have an overwhelming need for people to like/love/accept/approve of me.

_____ 19. I avoid making waves.

_____ 20. I go out of my way not to hurt people's feelings and end up being dishonest.

Okay, now that wasn't so hard, was it? If so, not to worry; you're only at the beginning of this book. You'll feel much better about yourself by the end of it. So here's how to score this little test. Give yourself 4 points for each *Always* answer, 3 for *Often*, 2 for *Sometimes*, and 1 for *Rarely/Never*, then add up your points. Now take a gander at the scores below and see where you fall:

60–80 Go make yourself a crown of thorns. You're killing yourself with kindness!

45–59 Find some thorns and get on the waiting list for a crown-making class.

25–44 Buy yourself a niceometer and monitor yourself extremely carefully.

20–24 Being too nice is not your problem.

Not to sound too much like a therapist, but how are you feeling about your score? Are you in shock? Did your answers reinforce what you'd already guessed about yourself? Are you so depressed you're considering drowning your sorrows in a milk shake?

All kidding aside, it's *tremendously* hard work to view yourself honestly and accept who you are—warts and all. And let's be real, being too nice is not the worst thing in the world. It's hardly up there with being an ax murderess or a mercenary. Take a deep breath and gently pull yourself out of self-flagellation mode and start courting curiosity. Hmm, so you're too nice, and that may be why you have an eating or weight problem. That's okay—you're smart, talented, a terrific problem solver (for other people, anyway), and you'll change and grow and be a finer femme for having done so.

▌**GRAB YOUR THINKING CAP** Look objectively at how you hurt yourself by being unilaterally nice. Can you recognize that this doesn't make you bad, but that you've merely taken a good thing too far? ▌

Could you be a tad more specific about what's wrong with me?

Before you can fix the problem, you have to recognize what it is and understand whence it came. Excessive niceness comes in many shapes and forms. You may have only some characteristics, or you may have the whole kit and caboodle. Because I'm a cognitive-behavioral therapist—I operate on the assumption that beliefs produce feelings and behavior and that changing beliefs transforms emotions and actions— I've divided up characteristics of the overly nice into three aspects of self: what you believe, what you feel, and how you behave. These examples will give you an idea of how too much niceness plays out; there are dozens more where they came from.

WHAT YOU BELIEVE

• I am responsible for people's happiness.

• I need to be upbeat and cheerful, and make people feel better.

• People will fall apart without my help.

• If I say what I feel, people will be hurt and won't like me.

• If I stop being overly nice, people won't accept me.

- I have to be perfect, including how I look and act and what I say.

- I need praise from others to feel okay about myself.

- Saying no to others' requests means I'm selfish.

- Putting myself first means I'm self-centered and don't care about others. *what is denying myself not saving self, etc.*

- I'm not a good person unless I'm being helpful or productive.

WHAT YOU FEEL

- I can't bear when people are in distress.

- I feel guilty letting people down by disappointing them or not meeting their needs.

- I feel driven to keep people's spirits up and to prevent them from suffering.

- I can't stand hurting people's feelings.

- I'm scared people won't like me if I stop being overly nice.

- I'm determined to be/look/act perfect because I hate failing or making mistakes.

- I feel inadequate and insecure unless people shower me with praise and compliments, although mostly I don't believe them.

• I hate the thought that I might be selfish and feel awful about myself when I think I am.

• I feel guilty if I take care of myself rather than other people.

• I feel lost and useless unless I'm doing something for others or being useful.

HOW YOU BEHAVE

• I listen endlessly to people's problems, offer solutions, and give advice.

• I do favors for people even when I don't have the time or the energy and they don't reciprocate.

• I'm a smiley face and cover my negative feelings to appear upbeat.

• I say things I don't mean and do things I don't want to do simply to avoid hurting someone's feelings.

• I avoid confronting and challenging people and am a yes-girl.

• I obsess about looking/acting/saying things perfectly and would rather die than make a mistake.

• I rarely stand up for myself, set and stick to clear and firm boundaries, or put myself first.

- Because I don't know when enough is enough, I overdo even when it stresses me to the max.

- Guilt drives most of my behavior and it's so automatic I don't even realize it.

- I don't know how to stop being so damed nice to people.

Are you starting to understand how what you believe and feel causes your nice button to be stuck in overdrive? And that your current thinking isn't doing you any favors? Face it: You're going to need a mental and emotional tune-up (maybe an entire rebuild, who knows?) to get your niceness factor into the healthy range. Still not convinced? Here are some examples that might pop open your eyes. Do any of these sound familiar?

- You spend so many hours on the phone at night helping your girlfriends solve their problems that you're too tired to do your laundry and go to work the next day wearing dirty clothes.

- You convince yourself that you can't make it to the gym because you're the only one who can finish that special project—the one that was begun by your coworkers who are all down at Mahoney's chugalugging their way through happy hour.

- Stressed out over the week from hell, you surround yourself with all your favorite foods and eat yourself into oblivion instead of calling a girlfriend and insisting that she zip her lip and let you rant and rave for five minutes.

want to be motivated by Love ...

1—1

- You say, "Sure, stay as long as you like," to out-of-town friends who suddenly appear on your doorstep when you've got the flu, and you sleep on the broken futon so they can enjoy your brand-new water bed.

- You constantly bolster your spouse's/partner's fragile ego so he or she won't fall into a pit of self-loathing and despair and, instead, become depressed yourself.

- You spend hours searching for just the right thing for your impossible-to-please parent's/sister's birthday, overnight it to him or her, never receive a thank-you, and go out and do the same thing the following year (and the one after that).

- You calculate that you've said "I'm sorry" seventeen times and it's only midday, although not one thing you apologized for was remotely your fault.

Okay, *now* you've got the picture and that blurry image of a too-nice person is getting clearer: Surprise, it's you! If you're feeling anxious or unsettled about this discovery, that's natural. Your mind is probably zooming ahead to how you're going to manage to get a nice-ectomy without losing too many friends—or your job. Well, stop right there. You aren't going to whip yourself into a made-over woman warrior in a week. This is not a crash diet—you already know those don't work.

Before you even start considering what to *do* about being too nice, you have to understand *how* and *why* you came to be the poster child for nicehood. Moreover, remember, you don't want to stop being nice completely. You just want to lop off some of that goodness and maybe bulk up other qualities—

selfishness, self-confidence, limit setting, candidness, and assertiveness—to round yourself out.

▮ **GRAB YOUR THINKING CAP** What is it like to reflect on specific beliefs, feelings, and behaviors that relate to niceness? Does this make you feel better or worse about yourself, or are your feelings a mixed bag? ▮

Was I born with twelve extra niceness genes or what?

It should come as no surprise that there's a big parental push for one of the genders to be "nice" while the other is encouraged to be everything else. Women are expected and socialized to be agreeable, pleasant, kind, comforting, nurturing, self-sacrificing, dependent, generous, good, polite, other-oriented, helpful, well behaved, gentle, sympathetic, compassionate, gracious, and, of course, respectful. There's nothing wrong with being any of these things—and many good reasons to cultivate such esteemed qualities—but flaunting them 24/7 makes you only half a healthy human being. If your intent is to *only* or *always* sport these traits, you elbow out the other essential qualities that will help you discover life's true sweet spots.

I won't go into a long historical account of how and why women have been jammed into the niceness slot, while men get to roam about and try out lots of different options to see what fits. Sure, women have made tremendous strides in cracking our nice shells and stepping out into the world more assured and empowered. However, it's hard to peel off a label that was stuck on at the beginning of human existence. It may be too late to change history, but it's never too late to change yourself.

However, it's not just history but also current culture—not only in the United States but all over the planet—that dangles the nice ideal in front of us and wags its finger when we aren't sweetie pies. While it's no longer the fifties, the error (oops, I mean era) in which I was brought up, when women were supposed to remove their aprons only to slip into their baby doll pajamas, we still have a long way to go not to be viewed as a bitch when we're outspoken and assertive. Even in this day and age, there are men (and sadly, women as well) telling us how we should and shouldn't act, what choices are okay to make and which ones will damn our souls to hell, and trying to narrow our rightful human potential.

Culture being what it is, we have two clear choices: to jump on the bandwagon or hijack it for our own purposes. I'm not looking to make you into a revolutionary. You may not care about equality between the sexes in general, and you may rather be mistaken for an ostrich than a feminista, but the fact is, if you blindly accept the female prescription to be nice at all costs, you may not be able to rid yourself of your eating problems and establish a comfortable weight. Let's remember that this book is about how putting yourself last drives you to food, which is another way of saying that being too nice can lead you to getting your face stuck in the cookie jar.

Gender aside, being good and caring is encouraged in school, through religion, on the playground, and just about everywhere else. It's a fine and necessary quality . . . as long as it doesn't apply to only one half of the species and doesn't crowd out every other personality card in the deck. There's nothing wrong with the Golden Rule, "Do unto others what you would have them do unto you." There's everything wrong with, "Do unto others and keep doing it in spite of the fact you never get done unto."

So it's the ways of the world that have done me wrong, right?

Not exactly. History is the backdrop for how we got to this point, and culture is our current stage, but there's much more going on. The most likely explanation for your over-niceness is how you were brought up, especially the role modeling done by your parents and, to a lesser degree, other relatives.

In an ideal family, you would have been raised to believe that, along with being nice, sometimes you have to risk being perceived as "naughty" to get what you want and deserve, and that sometimes you have to stop asking and simply grab what's rightfully yours. In more dysfunctional families (and whose isn't?), you're given erroneous, incomplete, or conflicting messages about niceness and caring about others. These messages generally skew to one extreme or the other: In dysfunctional families, parents often are either extremely giving or extremely selfish—and either extreme can send a kid into a too-nice tailspin.

Maybe everyone who ever met her said of your mother, "Oh, Marge, she's the nicest woman you'd ever want to know. What a saint!" Or perhaps she wasn't around much because she was working two jobs and you were raised by Grandma Flori or Aunt Juanita who were shining examples of piety and politeness. If your primary female role model avoided arguments, backed off from taking risks and challenges, fed off being praised, tried to keep the peace at all costs, couldn't stand to have people mad at her, kept quiet rather than said what was on her mind, took care of everyone but herself, or stressed herself out being Supermom or Superperson, well, small wonder you followed along in her saintly footsteps.

At the other extreme, your mother may have been mean, abusive, self-centered, a taker, or a not very warm and fuzzy human being, so that you vowed early on to be her opposite.

Now you're afraid that if you're not hypervigilant about keeping yourself on the nice wagon, you'll fall off and end up exactly like you know who. If you had one parent who was overly nice and one who was overly not nice, you may be wary of both options and confused about how to be. Or, maybe your parents ping-ponged between being nice one moment and nasty the next, so that you never learned there's an in-between. Perhaps neither of your parents treated you well, so you responded by keeping a low profile or yessing them to death. What else could you do? Rebelling would have risked more abuse, so you threw all your energy into desperately hoping that being extra good would drive away their meanness.

Just one more point about why you've spent most of your life angling to be Mother Teresa and I'll move on. When we're young, we think in the simplest terms. If we see only two positions, overly nice and not nice, with no gradient in between, we assume there are only two choices. We fear that if we pick overly nice, we'll be stepped on and run over, so we choose top dog over underdog. Or we select overly nice because it's unbearable to consider being not nice and hurting other people. A choice between a rock and a hard place if ever there was one. Who knew that there were other options? Not you.

▌ **GRAB YOUR THINKING CAP** From your upbringing, how were you programmed to be the nice queen? Are you trying to be like someone or unlike him or her, or are you confused about how to be? ▌

How can I ditch the nice girl persona and regain control of my eating?

Never fear—there's hope! By reading this book, you'll learn how putting yourself last and doing what others want rather than what *you* want has set you up to feel cheated and drives you to overeat. Of course, all the understanding in the world won't change you automatically, but insight leads to clearer, healthier thinking and forms the basis for making better decisions.

What you need is some balance in your life: to know when to say no and when to say yes, how to ask for help as easily as you give it, when to let other people live with the consequences of their choices, how to be honest with yourself (always) and forthright and direct with other people (most of the time), and why it's important to give up striving to be perfect and accept your perfectly imperfect self. Right about now, little voices in your head may be screaming that what I'm suggesting is too tall an order, that you'll never be able to succeed at scrubbing all that snowy whiteness out of you and allowing yourself a bit of tarnish. Or you may be terrified of uncovering some sourness or bitterness under that glossy, sugar-coated veneer.

All natural and normal reactions. Not to worry. I'm convinced that after reading this book you'll be able to reorder your priorities and reshuffle your goals, improve your relationship with food and be more comfortable in your body and, better yet, feel freer and more authentic than you've ever felt in your life.

NICE GIRL RECOVERY TIPS

- Add new, forceful personality traits—don't eliminate your niceness. Kindness, caring, consideration, and generosity are stellar qualities . . . as long as you don't go overboard with them and act in ways that are hurtful to yourself.

- Recognize that women have a history of subservience and are fighting an uphill battle to be not nice *and* accepted in today's society. Men don't have to jump through these hoops. If the deck seems stacked against you, it's because it is!

- Study women—past and present—who were courageous, outspoken, and powerful, and discover how they were able to succeed in spite of the fact that they weren't the nicest girls on the block. Use them as role models. All women need them.

- Talk to other women about the pressure to be nice. Think about starting a No More Nice Girls support group of friends, neighbors, or coworkers.

- Ask yourself how the roles of men and women in your family (particularly your parents) have shaped your desire to be so nice.

To do today

Catch yourself when you're about to apologize and instead say nothing!

Meet One of the Nice Girls

Mary now

Mary is a registered nurse in a large teaching hospital in Boston. Patients love her, colleagues sing her praises, and her supervisor says she can't imagine the mess her unit would be without her. Mary came to see me because a colleague had mentioned I work with women who overdo it, and this colleague kept nagging her until she made an appointment.

At forty-one, Mary continues to pour every ounce of her considerable skill and energy into being the best nurse she can be. If someone needs to switch shifts at the last minute, Mary'll do it; if there's an emergency on another floor, she's off to the rescue; if a patient or family member is especially difficult, she's by his or her side lending a hand. (I hope I have a nurse like her next time I'm in the hospital.)

Her husband is a quiet man, owner of a roofing company, who is nurturing and supportive, even more so since they lost an infant with a birth defect three years ago. The two are very close and spend much of their time outside work together, never straying far from home. Neither one likes to make waves and they're both self-confessed people pleasers. In fact, one of the reasons Mary is so well liked is that she finds it nearly impossible to say no. She knows why—"They won't like me"— but has only begun to explore the roots of her fears. Over time in therapy, on occasion, she's been able to say no to or challenge me, but when we began our work together, she agreed with everything I said or suggested no matter what her true feelings were.

Mary weighs nearly 275 pounds and recognizes that her eating problems are directly related to her inability to take better care of herself. However, she worries about keeping her job, patients being in pain and not properly cared for, making her fellow nurses spend extra time at work, "especially those with little ones." Being childless is her explanation for why she's willing to cut other nurses slack, but she admits that taking extra shifts is also her way of keeping her mind busy. Plus, she acknowledges that when she's asked to do something, even something she thinks might not be in her self-interest, it simply doesn't occur to her to refuse.

By her own admission, "My eating is abominable." She grabs food on the run, forgets about nutrition, waits until she's ravenous to eat, or goes in search of a snack when she has a minute to herself. Plan meals ahead? Never. She admits she doesn't really taste food or even care much what she's eating as long as it's easy to get, doesn't cost a fortune, and "isn't too far past the pull date." There's a definite gravitation to sweets and starchy snacks because, she insists, she needs energy to keep on trucking. Although she's tried dieting, she's never stuck to one for more than a few weeks, complaining that it's too hard. She jokes about her bad eating habits and doesn't seem to care about her weight. Because her husband is heavy and he's happy with her as she is, she lacks motivation to eat differently.

Mary as a child

She's the oldest of nine siblings, two of whom died before they reached their teens. Her mother was an LPN and her father spent most of his time and money drinking and complaining about being unemployed. She describes her mother as a "saint who did what she had to and didn't whine about it," and her father, well, the words aren't printable here! He was verbally and physically abusive when he was drunk and she and everyone else in the family steered clear of him. While her mother was at work, it was Mary's job to take care of the house and what she calls "the brood." She didn't have to be asked twice to do something and tried to be a clairvoyant and anticipate everyone else's needs and wishes. When I asked what she did in her free time, she looked at me as if I were crazy.

Rarely did she complain to her mother, whom she didn't want to burden. She just kept putting one foot in front of the other until she left home to marry after completing nursing school. She avoided challenging her father on any fronts because she was afraid he'd go after her, watching in terror as her more rebellious siblings got knocked around. If she didn't do her best with "the brood," she feared letting down her mother and angering her father. Interestingly, she was thin until she got married. "All that running around," she told me, "who had time to eat?"

De-nicing Mary

Mary has been a bit of a challenge, in part because she isn't terribly motivated to do the hard work of therapy nor is she consciously unhappy with her life. I told her right off that I saw a number of issues for her to work on: eating, an inability to say no, and a need to grieve for her deceased child. To say that Mary is not eager to work on any of these issues is an understatement, but she manages to stay engaged in therapy enough to make some inroads without ever admitting she needs and values the help.

On the eating front, I ask her to keep a food diary, something I rarely do because most of the women I see already focus too much on food. But Mary needs to stop and think about food, and when she reads over her diary, she's appalled at what she puts into her mouth. Instead of encouraging her to regulate her eating, I encourage her to pick nutritious substitutes when she wants to eat, whether from hunger or stress. This is not as hard as Mary has feared, and she's surprised she has more energy when she eats more healthily.

Much of the therapy focuses on her childhood: the burden of being a parentified child with overwhelming responsibility at too young an age and dealing with her passive mother and abusive, alcoholic father. This work takes a long time, but slowly Mary discovers that saying no to doing a double shift won't close the hospital and that leaving work on time can make her feel proud, not ashamed. Her first major step in the self-care direction is to take a weekly yoga class. We also talk a lot about the loss of her child, and this is a pivotal point in the therapy. She even brings her husband in for a few sessions so that they can grieve together, and Mary begins changing in spite of herself.

What's Next? *In Chapter 2, "Using Food as Self-Care," you'll learn*

• About the biology of eating and weight

• How stress makes you eat

• How personality traits push you toward food and away from people

TWO

Doesn't Everyone's Best Friend Live in Her Refrigerator?

Using Food as Self-Care

Why food? you might ask. Of all the possible best friends in this world, why pick something that has to be trucked in, costs a mint, and might rot before its pull date? For that matter, why choose something that even *has* a pull date. Why not go along with the song and make diamonds your best friend? Or your dog? Strange as it seems, there are actually some odd ducks out there who believe that friendship makes for better self-care than food. If so, why go for the goodies rather than a gab with the gals?

One reason we choose food over friends is that unless you live in a commune, it's unlikely that your buddies are as close as your refrigerator. You choose edibles over practically everything else that has the potential to make you feel better because it's accessible. Never mind reaching out and touching someone; it's easier to walk a few paces in any direction and swallow some comfort or drive a couple of blocks and indulge in dietary distraction.

Another reason you head for the refrigerator when the phone (if we're measuring actual distance here) might be closer is that food is never too busy to be eaten; it's not off skiing in Switzerland or spending the afternoon at the mall getting the kids new sneakers. It never has emergencies or gets snooty when you want it to shut up and listen. It has no agenda of its own and no needs except to disappear while making you blissfully, deliriously happy.

And, oh, can food make you swoon! A friend may give you a there-there pat on the back or a heart-to-heart hug, she may turn your blubbering into a giggle fit with some goofy insight that pops things back to perspective, or sling some snarky remark your way to snap you back to reality. She may even suck out the poison of some awful sting of emotion. But all that only brings you back to normal. Food catapults you over the moon and beyond with how yummy it feels in your mouth, on your tongue, going down, in your tummy. It's like a swami's carpet, winging you to Fantasy Island where everything's right and nothing is wrong. People are mere mortals; food is divine.

Food is as familiar as that stuffed animal you can't throw away and keep handy for those moments when nothing else will do. There's no thinking involved when you grab for it, no surprises. Just knowing food is there lightens your load and brightens your day. It's satisfaction guaranteed because that's how it's always been . . . or has been for so long you can't remember a time when food was simply something you ate when you were hungry. We are creatures of habit who long for security and certainty, especially when we're blue. If that security is topped with a flaky crust or sprinkled with confectioners' sugar that melts in your mouth, all the better.

More important than all of this is the fact that, to most of us, food equals love. Love is often what you crave when hunger is the last thing on your mind and food is the first thing in your mouth. How do you know food is love? Well, golly, haven't you gotten that message since you were barely larger than a bread box? Have a lollipop, try a cupcake, I made it just for you, but this is your favorite dessert, I know you never eat white food but I couldn't resist whipping this up for your special occasion, have some and you'll feel better, just taste it for me. How often when you wanted an arm around you did you instead get an outstretched hand with food in it? For many of us, food was a poor substitute, but it was better than nothing.

From the moment we see or hear our first food commercial, we're brainwashed into equating food with love. Some of you may be too young to remember the Pillsbury Doughboy and "Nothin' says lovin' like something from the oven." No subtlety there. What the Pillsbury folks were preaching is that food is conceived in love and that we'll feel a whole lot more of it when we partake of their goodies. Of course, when you stop and think about it, the message is ludicrous: Their breads and cookies are made in sterile vats by machines, baked in enormous ovens, shipped in trucks, and stored on supermarket shelves all by people who are hardly in love with what they're doing or the product they're selling . . . or you. But they need not be; the message goes straight to our hearts.

How 'bout the role of eating in celebrations and festivities? Throughout the ages, food has been a way to signify bonding and making merry. Breaking bread cemented the peace by bringing warring tribes together after bloody battles. In olden times, people offered each other food to show they meant no harm, as a way to wangle themselves into each other's good graces, and to mark special occasions (remember, there were no gift cards back then). Women gathered food together, men hunted in packs, and at the end of the day, they sat around the fire feeding their empty bellies, feeling pride in their joint efforts and enjoying the communal spirit (and often the communal spirits, as well).

If I throw out my TV, join a commune, and avoid parties, will I stop worshipping in my pantry?

Sorry, no. One of the primary reasons we cozy up to food when we're feeling icky or out of whack is that the drive to eat is built into our biology and reinforced by our earliest experiences. Think about our intro to food. As infants, feeding takes up a preponderance of time on our limited social calendars. But it's not just the feeding that rings our chimes. Sure, we need sustenance or we'll die. It's what happens while we're being fed. The fortunate among us are held while we're enjoying our lactose fix, whether it's formula or the real deal. Nestled in loving arms, we're cooed at and stroked while sucking ourselves into oblivion. The tryptophan in milk provides a chemical cocktail that causes us to relax and feel drowsy, and we automatically begin to associate feeding with feeling satisfied, comforted, and soothed. Picture it: We awaken in distress, bawling our tiny hearts out for food, are held and fed, and return to slumber. Heaven, did someone say heaven?

When this interaction is repeated hundreds of times over the course of infancy, through a process called conditioning we naturally come to associate feeding with the alleviation of internal distress. The fact that food tastes good makes us want to eat it because of how our brain's pleasure center responds. In layperson's language, treats (foods high in sugar and fat) tend to make our gray matter light up like a Fourth of July celebration. We respond positively to treats (a stimulus) and remember our reaction (a response), so that we seek out the conditions under which we may encounter it again and again. Eventually the response becomes a reflex, which drives the desire for the stimuli.

treat >> pleasure in brain >> seek treat >> pleasure in brain

On the other hand, for those whose chief cook and bottle washer was Mommy Dearest, feedings might have felt more like bondage than bonding. Maybe Mom handled us roughly and was out of sync with our needs, shoving a bottle into our clamped lips or painfully yanking it away before we were satisfied. Maybe she was sick, too depressed, busy, tired, or uninterested to spend much time nourishing and cuddling our infant selves. Perhaps there were too many birds in her nest and feeding us was a mere pit stop on the way to other obligations. If there was no daddy around to help or only Daddy Dearest, she may have done the best she could, but that best was far from good enough.

If our infant anguish was intense enough, it eventually may have turned into despair and paved the way for the unconscious belief that *nothing* would make us feel better. If our hungers (for food, touch, or calming) weren't attended to in a timely and loving manner, we may have suffered such acute emotional and physical distress that not being soothed became encoded in our memories as an avoid-at-all-cost experience. Can you see what's happening here? We learned that what we felt was intolerable, that we are inconsolable, and we therefore hung a big "don't go there" sign on our brain that flashes at the first sign of distress.

While some of us began our lives learning to associate food with feeling better, others didn't discover until childhood or adolescence that food was the perfect elixir for emotional pain. Maybe our parents took potshots at each other at the dinner table and it was more comfortable to keep spooning those mashed potatoes onto our plate and shoving them into our mouth than listen to their shouting match. Perhaps they overtly favored a sibling or constantly berated us, so we ran off to our bedroom with a box of Pepperidge Farm Soft Baked cookies hidden under our shirt to take the edge off our hurt. Unconsciously the process went something like this: Food or pain? Pain or food? Duh!

■ **GRAB YOUR THINKING CAP** Describe your relationship with food in childhood and adolescence. Do you know anything about your earliest feedings that would explain your dysfunctional attachment to food today? ■

How come I'd pick tiramisù over tofu any day of the week?

Because you're no dummy. You've already figured out that all foods aren't created equal when it comes to making us feel better. Which leads me to the reason we choose treats to brighten a dark mood or smooth out life's rough spots: The chemical properties of certain edibles actually change our chemistry (remember milk making us feel drowsy as infants?). Steamed broccoli and broiled cod are not on the feel-good-now food list. They're not what you crave when you're marooned on misery island, are so jacked up you can't sit still, or feel as if your brains are about to fall out. That's when you'd kill for a Ring Ding, some gooey fudge, banana cream pie, pizza, macaroni and cheese, Reese's Pieces, and anything else made with spoonfuls of sugar and gobs of fat.

These cravings make you feel a little crazy (okay, more than a little) because you know you're trying to do the straight and narrow thing with food, but you simply cannot help yourself. It feels like invasion of the body snatchers; staring back at you in the mirror is Dr. Jekyll *and* Ms. Hyde. The problem is physical, not mental. Here's what's going on. There are brain and hormonal substances that impact our desire for food and, in fact, dictate our cravings for carbohydrates. One of them is cortisol, a hormone the brain produces as an anesthetic for pain. In response to tension and stress, our adrenal glands automatically produce excess cortisol that, in turn, stimulates a brain chemical called neuropeptide Y. Think of this little guy as in charge of the switch that turns carbo cravings on and off.

Still with me? Here's the path you follow without even realizing it:

tension >> excess cortisol >> neuropeptide Y >> carb craving

All these interactions occur automatically on a cellular level. You don't ask neuropeptide Y for help; he just gives it to you because he thinks it's his job to protect you from emotional pain. The problem is that when we consume more carbohydrates than our body needs, especially those that are high fat, they are converted into body fat. The real kick in the butt is that these tension-generating chemicals also make the body hold on to the new body fat. Talk about a double whammy.

As if that news isn't bad enough, it turns out that carbohydrates trigger a chemical reaction that increases the production of serotonin, a neurotransmitter (a chemical messenger that helps relay signals from one area of the brain to another) generally viewed as an emotional relaxant. Tension and stress deplete and lower serotonin levels so that you crave carbohydrates to raise them back up, that is, so you'll feel better. Here's the path this process follows:

tension >> decrease in serotonin >> carbs >>
increase in serotonin

Are you getting why we call certain yummies "comfort food"? They actually do, on a physiological level, relieve us of stress and help us feel better. On a Friday night, after the week from hell, you're not out of your mind when you bypass that healthy, balanced meal you steamed with the organic produce you paid a fortune for and instead dive headfirst into the left-over linguini Alfredo that's probably a day's worth of calories and then some. You wan't relief from stress and, hey, it's just a swallow away.

Okay, now, I'm not trying to turn any of you into winners of the Nobel Prize in biochemistry. But I do need to answer the question that began this chapter: why food so easily becomes a girl's best friend, especially if she's a nice girl. The answer is that by being so nice—so caring, giving, generous to a fault, self-effacing, responsible, and other-oriented—you put enor-mous pressure on yourself, which stresses you out whether you realize it or not. By not taking care of yourself in healthy, effective ways, you end up using food as your primary com-fort, and this behavior reinforces itself every time you reach for food when you're not hungry.

▌ **GRAB YOUR THINKING CAP** Do you feel any relief knowing that it makes perfect biological sense for you to turn to food for comfort? ▌

If I'm programmed to eat comfort foods when I'm stressed, is being overweight my destiny?

Although scientific studies tell us that some 50 to 70 percent of our weight is genetically determined,[1] please don't think you're stuck in fat jail with no means of escape. That statistic means that 30 to 50 percent of what you weigh *is* under your control, assuming you're willing to take the reins and make sensible, healthy lifestyle choices that will make it easier for you to eat "normally." By the way, "normal" eating is based on four simple rules: Eat when you're hungry, make satisfying food choices, eat consciously and with enjoyment, and stop eating when full or satisfied.

We've talked about the general reasons you overeat or eat when you're not hungry—biochemistry, cultural norms, and family socialization—so now it's time to zero in on the specifics of how you get into trouble with food because of your niceness. By recognizing that what you've considered a sterling virtue all these decades is, in the extreme, actually a vice that sabotages your health, you'll start to see what behaviors to change to kick the habit! Please remember, most of these patterns are so automatic and ingrained that you don't even realize you're stabbing yourself in the back with your nice wand every time you try to use it.

You don't like to "burden" others

In spite of the umpteen hours you spend listening to family and friends ranting and raving while wracking your brain for solutions and spreading nice balm all over their emotional wounds, in spite of how you're always there for others and ask but little of their time to help you, somehow when you think about taking five minutes to complain, you feel guilty about asking for too much. Never mind that your husband just took off to Acapulco with your best friend, your boss gave you your walking papers, or your child got arrested for selling drugs in school. When your sister calls to see how you are, you chirp, "Just fine, thanks, and you?"

"Fine" is your favorite word and you use it to death. I can't tell you how many times I've had women (on occasion, men too) enter my office looking as if they've just been run over by a bus respond to my asking how they're doing with "fine." Excuse me? Fine? *I* know they're not and *they* know they're not, but it's like pulling teeth to get their mouth to form any other word. They're like the dolls that talk when you pull the string, except these dolls have only one response: fine.

❙❙ **GRAB YOUR THINKING CAP** Have you told someone today that you were fine when in truth you were anything but? ❙❙

Let's talk about why you're addicted to saying you're fine when clearly you're not. Maybe you think no one cares if your life is in shambles. Most likely your experience early in life was that your feelings were ignored or minimized. If everyone at the dinner table got to yap their heads off about their day, but the dishes were whisked away before you had your turn, you might believe that your feelings don't count. If you had a sibling who was showered with attention (because she had a childhood disease or he was simply a pain-in-the-butt attention seeker), you probably got the message that other people deserve to spend their life in the spotlight but that you need to wait silently in the wings. I had a client whose father would make her leave the dinner table when she started to cry, even as a young child, while teasingly calling her Sarah Bernhardt. (For you youngsters, Ms. Bernhardt was a famous French actress in the late 1800s who was known for starring in melodramatic tragedies.) The message this father was telling his daughter was to stop overdramatizing—even when she wasn't. The subtext of the message is: You're just a drama queen and no one wants to listen to you.

Not wanting to "burden" others with your troubles, though, is a special kind of unwillingness to share your emotions. What you fear is that your feelings are unnatural and too much for others to bear or help you with, that you're oversensitive (a favorite pejorative word of parents), that what's going on within you (that you have the nerve to wish to express) is over the top, so kindly turn off the spiggot. Somewhere along the line you bought into the myth that your feelings were too big for other people, while the truth is that *the people* were too small (emotionally) to handle them—that is, your caretakers simply weren't up to the task. Whatever the reason, you grew up thinking that your natural feelings are burdensome to others. Wrong, wrong, and wrong again!

Another way you might have come to believe it's wrong to "burden" others is if someone in your family was a burden on you. You know what it feels like to carry and bear more than your share, and you're empathic enough not to want to inflict that load on others. You might have had to listen to your alcoholic father blather through monologues of self-recrimination when you wanted to finish your algebra homework or go to bed. You might have been a captive audience when your mother forced you to listen in excruciating detail to the miseries of her marriage or the travesties of her life. She might have acted as if you were her best friend or confessor, treating you as an adult when you were only a little bit of a thing. You may have vowed never to burden others as you were unfairly burdened.

Yes, some folks do go on and on about the minutiae of their lives. But those people are not you! These people not only don't fear that they're burdening others, it would never even occur to them that they are. In my considerable experience, folks who are burdensome generally have no clue that our eyes are glazing over as we listen (or try to avoid listening) to them, and it would truly shock them to learn that we aren't hanging on their every word.

■ **GRAB YOUR THINKING CAP** Do you really yack so much about your problems that you burden other people, or is this judgment all in your head? Have you ever asked? ▮

You don't pick people who can take care of you well emotionally

At the other end of the spectrum from women who are the Queen of Nice are those who are Queen of Ice. Yes, there are Kings of Nice and Ice, too. If I had my way, all the Kings and Queens of Nice would form a club and hang out exclusively together, but all you kindhearted souls out there won't let that happen. Instead, you pair up with and befriend people who are anywhere from slightly to shockingly coldhearted in the hopes of warming them up. Such is life that opposites attract. When you should be surrounding yourself with intimates who provide a gloriously mutually satisfying relationship—you talk, I listen and I talk, you listen—you find people who are all mouth and no ears.

Because you're afraid of burdening people, you keep mum about your troubles and are a superb listener. So naturally, someone wanting an audience or a soapbox finds you the perfect match. An emotionally healthy person recognizes that it's as important to share feelings as it is to listen to other people share theirs. An overly nice person, however, often finds her other half in someone who can only spout off. There is a natural attraction between opposites, because each represents half a balanced person, in this case the burdenee (you) and the burdener (them).

Unfortunately, unless you understand this complicated dynamic (called projection or sometimes projective identification), you're likely to choose friends who don't support you emotionally, reinforcing your belief that you're a—anyone want to guess?—"burden." I can almost guarantee that as a nice person you're highly unlikely to trouble others with your problems, but I'll stake my reputation that you've got a lot of people in your intimate circle who don't think twice about crying on your shoulder. Do you spend a lot of time wondering why people don't listen when you (on rare occasion) venture to bring up your difficulties? This crazy-making, unhealthy situation can lead you straight down the supermarket aisle and directly to the checkout counter with a cartload full of sugar and saturated fat.

▌ **GRAB YOUR THINKING CAP** Name three people you can count on to take care of you emotionally, no matter what. How many of your relationships are based on emotional mutuality? ▌

You're more comfortable being a caregiver than being taken care of

Although your secret dream may be to shrug off the heavy mantle of your private sorrows, to live lightly and effortlessly, and to give over all responsibility for taking care of you to someone else . . . strangely, the opposite happens more often than not. You may think you've found that perfect someone to take care of you—he brings flowers and takes you for candlelight dinners, she treats you to the movies and calls you five times a day to remind you you're her best friend—but slowly the relationship shifts and becomes like most of the others you've had: You do most of the heavy lifting. You may shake your head in amazement, recalling the good old days when you were certain you were finally going to have your needs heard and met, and now you spend hours wondering what you did wrong for the tables to have turned.

What you did wrong is choose people who are unable to take care of you emotionally. Not only do you fit together like a hand in a glove, but each of you gets to do what is most comfortable. Although you may desperately yearn to lay down your load, quite frankly, you're used to shouldering it. Maybe you believe that asking for help means you're weak or incapable, or you're convinced that no one can take care of you like you can. These untruths are born of your experience, but they don't hold water today. If you want to be taken care of, you'll have to stretch out of your usual role and be uncomfortable.

You're too busy taking care of other people to take care of yourself

If you're paying bills for the blind lady who lives next door, have volunteered to pick up the slack for your colleague who's out on maternity leave, agreed to chair this year's For the Cure walkathon in your community, and promised your son to make a quilt for your grandchild-to-be, when in heaven's name do you think you're going to have time to kick back and relax? Being nice takes time. Caring for yourself takes time. We get twenty-four hours only every day. Do the math: If your whole day is spent doing for others, you have little or no time left over for yourself.

I know what you say to yourself because I've heard it all before: I should go to the gym/take a walk/rest a little/read a book/go to sleep/get a haircut/book a massage/meditate/make a doctor's appointment/go on vacation. You reprimand yourself for not doing these things as you're racing out the door to take part in the neighborhood cleanup, head in to work on your day off, take chicken soup to a sick friend, or pick up your mother from the airport at 6 A.M. because she was thrilled she could get such a cheap flight.

Hello. These activities are not self-care. You might as well be beating yourself with a wire hairbrush. These gifts you bestow on others are the one-two (and ten-eleven) punch that knocks you down and keeps you out for the count. These little giving sprees eat up your time and energy so that all you're left with is exhaustion, a splitting headache, and a Snickers wrapper. Remember, in your mind, there's always time to eat. A candy bar is a quicker picker-upper than a twenty-minute, feet up sit-down with your eyes closed in an easy chair. A burger and fries inhaled on the way to pick up your husband's dry cleaning, which he forgot to get, are so much less effort than a home-made lunch and a walk in the park. Leftover tuna casserole gobbled at the stove is so much easier than telling your child that she's going to have to wait a few minutes and may be late to meet her friends at the mall because you need time to finish dinner sitting down. Need I go on?

▌ **GRAB YOUR THINKING CAP** When was the last time you said no to a request, set a limit and held to it, let someone be put out who wasn't you? ▐

You don't like feeling uncomfortable emotions

As a certified nice person, it makes sense that you enjoy ex-periencing only pleasant emotions. You love loving, feeling loved and valued, being kind, nonjudgmental, open-minded, empathic, giving, caring, supportive, and generous. These emo-tions lead to other good feelings, especially pride. Feeling angry, conflicted, judgmental, selfish, and disappointed in others is not your cup of tea. These emotions are not only yucky, but you may consider them "bad." You believe they're bad because they make you feel bad (that is, unhappy, distressed, etc.). You're confusing the discomfort of the affective state (the emo-tion) and your displeasure at having it, which is called feeling bad about feeling bad.

In all likelihood, you were brought up to think that having (or expressing) negative emotions makes you a "bad" person. Now hear this: You are not bad because you have negative feelings.

You're normal! There are no such things as "good" and "bad" feelings; all emotions are fair game and natural. Emotions, like musical notes and colors, are value neutral. We need 'em all to paint a picture and create a symphony. People who do horrible things (folks we might think of as "bad" people) have nice feelings, and nice people have horrible feelings. Now, isn't that a relief?

That doesn't mean that uncomfortable, painful, or negative feelings are a day at the beach. Grief is heart-wrenching, betrayal can pull the rug right out from under you, rage can make you feel as if you're about to expode, and confusion can make your head spin. The key to emotional management is the way you view emotions. If you think of them as scary, unsettling, overwhelming, debilitating, and nasty—who wants to dwell on painful things, anyway?—you're going to want to run from them (and, more than likely, toward food).

On the other hand, if you view emotions as necessary, manageable, informative, interesting, and a natural part of life, you'll be curious about them and let them visit as they please (within reason). When you're comfortable with any and all emotions, you understand that you don't become Freddy Krueger just because you're angry, that you don't turn into an ungrateful witch because you refuse to be taken advantage of and set limits, and that you aren't a meanie because you won't buy your kids every toy in Toy World.

And, surprise, when you view emotions this way, you don't turn to food to distract yourself from inner turmoil.

▌ **GRAB YOUR THINKING CAP** Quick, three words that describe how you feel about having uncomfortable, painful, distressing emotions. ▌

Is it possible for me to perform a nice-ectomy on myself?

I understand that you may be freaking out and despairing that you're stuck with your niceness (and excess weight) forever. You're bummed because what you thought was your best quality is turning out to be your worst, or at least the one that's causing you to overeat. Fear not. You don't have to become the Wicked Witch of the West in order to have a comfortable relationship with food. You do, however, have to acquire more effective self-care and emotional management skills, which is far easier than quantum physics but substantially harder than blowing out all your birthday candles.

You'll need to think and act differently and expand your self-care repertoire (making a choice between peanut brittle and Cheez Doodles is not a repertoire) to stop seeking comfort in food. A word here about change. Change is hard, change takes time, but thinking about it in terms of acquiring skills makes it easier. All my books about eating and weight use a skills-based approach. Skills are behaviors learned with practice and patience. You simply start out with no or minimal skills and you keep at it until you know what you're doing. Anyone can learn skills. There's nothing magical and mystical about them. After all, you learned to eat and be nice.

NICE GIRL RECOVERY TIPS

• Ask yourself why you turn to food when you're in emotional distress. The urge is not all in your head. Refuse to be hard on yourself when you eat when you're not hungry or overeat. Cultivate compassion and curiosity!

- Learn more about stress, eating, weight, and biology—not to become a biochemist but to develop a better understanding of the role biochemistry and heredity play in stress and eating.

- Reread the personality traits described in this chapter. As you read them slowly for a second time, notice if you respond to them differently. Maybe you didn't see yourself the first time or maybe you did and felt angry but now feel some compassion.

- Ask yourself which personality traits plague you and cause you to be overly nice. Don't obsess about changing them or devise a plan to obliterate them, just muse about how they affect you and notice what feelings and thoughts surface.

- Ask yourself why you're afraid of letting go of being so nice. Reassure yourself that you won't become an ogre, but will learn to temper your niceness with other positive traits.

- Consider how you generally view emotions and how you will have to change your perspective to become healthier emotionally and around food.

To do today

Risk burdening another person by talking about a problem that troubles you.

Meet One of the Nice Girls

Rosa now

Rosa is thirty years old, single, and a teacher's aide, attending night school to obtain a degree in elementary education. She's a second-generation Peruvian American, an incredibly hard worker who takes on every task her supervising teacher asks. Although she loves working with children, she finds the demands of the school system stressful because she worries about following the rules and not getting into trouble. Cordial with colleagues, she keeps her distance and never feels part of the group, a problem she's had since childhood, which she attributes to her family's immigrant status.

At some sixty pounds overweight, Rosa feels rotten about herself and is anxious about damaging her health. She jokingly wishes she could be like some people and deny her eating and weight problems. Rosa says she's an emotional eater who turns to food to prevent herself from feeling distress or to soothe herself when uncomfortable feelings start to overwhelm her. She adores carbohydrates and sweets and has stashes of goodies in her purse, car, classroom closet, and all over her apartment.

Rosa has a few close friends but no romantic relationship, although she says she's eager to find someone to settle down with. She desperately wants to have children and worries she's already "over the hill." The one long-term relationship she had at twenty-four was a disaster. Her boyfriend was emotionally and physically abusive and she left him only when her family intervened and threatened to report him to the police. Since then, Rosa has barely dated because she's afraid she'll pick another hothead. She mistrusts her judgment in general and is especially self-doubting around men and food.

Rosa as a child

Rosa's parents—her mother is a doctor and her father an architect—are from Peru and sent her here when she was nine to live with her maternal grandmother until they could bring over her three younger siblings. Rosa hated being separated from her family and cried for a month when she moved in with her widowed grandmother, who took good physical care of her but simply was not tuned in to a child's needs. A new neighborhood, school, and culture intimated Rosa, and her grandmother was no help, as she herself hadn't mastered English and didn't push herself to assimilate.

Her grandmother's best efforts to care for Rosa came through food. She was an excellent cook and loved to watch her granddaughter eat—and eat—the native dishes she made for her. Rosa describes her grandmother as literally standing over her at mealtime ladling soup into her bowl or scooping stew onto her plate the minute she finished a helping. Although there were plenty of rules living with her grandmother, Rosa could eat as much as she wanted whenever she wanted.

By the time her parents arrived in this country, Rosa was ten and overjoyed to see them and her siblings. Her parents bought a large house in an upscale neighborhood in the town next to her grandmother, so once more Rosa had to change schools and make new friends. Her parents pressured her to do well academically and measure up to American standards, pushing her to "make something of myself." The harder she tried, however, the lower her grades dropped, until she didn't even want to attend school. Her parents insisted she see the school counselor, where Rosa finally was able to talk about not fitting in, never measuring up to expectations, and not knowing how both to be true to herself and please others.

De-nicing Rosa

Rosa's experience is fairly typical of immigrant children from professional homes where education and excelling are highly prized. Our discussions about her fears and wishes helped her relax and explore what she really wanted out of life. Unlike her parents, she had no desire to become a "professional" anything; she only wanted to support herself and have a respectable job. More than that, she wanted a family. We discussed how her parents' expectations affected her growing up and how having chosen the wrong man and retreating from dating have prevented her from reaching her goals.

We also explored how her frustrated yearnings get translated into dysfunctional eating. While she's eating she doesn't worry about not fitting in, disappointing her parents, feeling undervalued by her supervising teacher, and not having a boyfriend. She immediately made the connection to using food to cope the same way she did when she lived with her grandmother. We focused on the steps she needs to take to experience her distress so that she can find her way out of it, including tolerating letting down her folks, speaking up when she feels undervalued and overworked, and risking putting herself out there to start dating.

What's Next? In Chapter 3, "Finding Substitutes to Eating," you'll learn

- The definitions of life skills and self-care strategies

- The life skills that are essential to happiness, success, reducing stress, and maximizing your potential

- The self-care strategies that will help you manage emotions effectively and avoid abusing food

THREE

If It Doesn't Have Frosting, What Good Is It?

Finding Substitutes to Eating

Funny how life works. It just so happens that the attitudinal and behavioral shifts you need to make to eliminate unwanted eating are the exact changes necessary to put the brakes on excessive niceness. So you actually get two prizes for the price of one. I'm not going to soft-pedal the work that must be done. Shedding some of your kindness and caring and finding new ways to act is a herculean feat, but it's absolutely, definitely doable. You won't transform yourself overnight and new behaviors will not necessarily generate immediate happiness. In fact, you might feel a lot worse before you feel better. But if life is more pits than cherries, what do you have to lose (but weight)?

Many of you, though champing at the bit to begin your

emotional makeover, may be clueless about how to make it happen. Perhaps you have a vague idea that you really ought to stop volunteering for thankless tasks or get to the gym more often, but beyond that, it's all a blur. Fortunately, there are tried-and-true ways to both de-nice yourself and curb unwanted eating. Specifically, you need to build life skills and develop healthy self-care strategies. *Life skills* are basic tools for living, the general abilities required to negotiate the world successfully. *Self-care strategies* are the behaviors and activities necessary to keep yourself in good running order—physically, mentally, and emotionally.

These skills and strategies are nothing like studying math or grammar; you can't hunker down and simply memorize them. Learning is gradual, and you have to keep practicing or you'll lose the knack. In fact, you can read all the self-help books in the world and go to self-esteem workshops day and night, and it won't make a darned bit of difference if you're not willing to roll up your sleeves and do the muscle-building work of self-renovation. Building life skills and developing self-care strategies are part of experiential learning, which means stretching yourself and gradually growing into a healthier person.

A reminder for all you speed demons that change always happens far too slowly for our liking. Wanting it yesterday and not getting it for many, many tomorrows is a frustrating and maddening process. You have to keep your eyes riveted to your goals, learn from your mistakes, and avoid comparing yourself to others. Everyone starts out at a different place in life; therefore, some people find change easier than others. Actually, forget easy altogether. If transformation were simple and effortless, you wouldn't be reading this book and I wouldn't have written it!

Enough said. It's time to learn the steps that will cut the emo-

ıal cord between you and food and discover the path that will
lead you out of Niceville. What follows is a description of skills
you need to master. Not today or by the end of the week. Not
even this year. They're called *life* skills not only because they help
you manage out there but also because you (and everyone else)
will spend your entire existence honing them.

Life skills to learn

Identify, express, and manage feelings

You're used to tuning out what you really feel, ignoring or
minimizing your needs, swallowing your words, and letting
people run roughshod over you (not to mention stuffing your
face to avoid distress). You may not even know what you feel
or need to make you happy. Many of my clients are dumb-
founded when I ask them what they're feeling. They haven't a
clue. The emotions you're most in touch with are likely guilt,
shame, regret, and frustration. Or maybe resentment. Or feeling insecure and overwhelmed. Or perhaps a simmering, underlying rage you call stress.

Well, now hear this: Emotions are your inner guide to the
outer world. You do no one any good if you're emotionally dishonest with yourself. Emotions make themselves known one
way or the other. They have a habit of sneaking up or leaking
out even when you try your best to squelch them—*especially*
when you try to squelch them. You don't have to act on every
emotion, but it is essential that you know exactly what you're
feeling 24/7. Yikes, you're saying, every minute of every day?
In a word, yes. Maybe you won't know in the moment and will
need time to reflect until you recognize, *Aha*, that's *what I was
feeling*. Not a problem. Just remember, the goal is to keep tabs
on your heart.

Of course, first you have to recognize and acknowledge that

you have an uncomfortable feeling, that the knot in your stomach isn't from the pizza with extra anchovies or the moo shoo shrimp. Then it's time to identify the precise feeling—disappointment, betrayal, rage, guilt, shame, etc. Dig down under "bad," "upset," and "hurt"; they're way too general to be helpful. The more exact the identification, the greater your understanding.

You also need to express emotions openly and directly. Twenty questions and charades are fun party games, but they don't work with feelings. No one should have to guess your mood or desires. Sure, your mouth is for eating, but it's also for putting what's in your mind and heart out into the world. Learning to communicate directly and effectively is not optional. If you want a better relationship with yourself and others (and food), it's a must. You also need to figure out how to experience and tolerate uncomfortable affect when immediate expression isn't in your best interest, say, when your jerk of a boss accidentally rubs up against you seductively when you're with a client. You'd like to clobber him one, but really, where will *that* get you? Self-care strategies, which you'll hear more about later in this chapter, will help you learn how to contain affect and soothe distress.

If you're not adept at acknowledging and identifying feelings, stop chasing your tail and get help—read self-help books, find a therapist, or join a group where emotional pain and suffering are openly explored. By the way, the reason emotional management is life skill numero uno is that it's essential to curbing both your niceness and your appetite and to developing other life skills.

▌GRAB YOUR THNKING CAP Which of the following are difficult for you to do? Experience discomfort or pain? Identify emotions? Express feelings? Soothe your distress? ▌

Establish and maintain boundaries

Most children know about not crossing a line from playing games. So how come you don't? Remember as a kid when you weren't supposed to step over a certain boundary? Well, fast-forward a couple of decades and notice how you let your life blend into someone else's until you've almost disappeared, how you allow people to wander over the border and invade your territory. What happened? There are two possibilities: Either you didn't set boundaries to begin with, or you're not enforcing them.

Setting and maintaining boundaries is necessary for navigating through any network—family, friends, work, community. Roles need not be rigid and lines can shift when necessary, but basically *you* get to decide where your limits are; you don't hand the decision making over to someone else. You make up your mind what you can and cannot do and then stick to your guns no matter who tries to guilt-trip, wheedle, bully, shame, or nag you into changing your mind. You have to be strong about setting limits and rigid about enforcing them. Initially folks will test whether you're serious. When they know you are, they'll be more likely to honor your boundaries. Sure, sometimes they'll need a gentle reminder; other times they'll need numerous ungentle reminders. Either way, *you're* the crossing guard, so act like one.

▌▌ **GRAB YOUR THINKING CAP** Why are you afraid to set and enforce boundaries? ▌▌

Separate effectively from family and become autonomous

When people look at you, do they see your mother or father? No, they see you, a unique individual unlike any other now or ever. So how come there's confusion at your folks' house? Mom gets cold and insists you need a sweater. Dad, aka Mr.

Math, keeps pressing you about joining his accounting firm when you have to take off your shoes and socks to count. Grandma, who married late, insists that what you need to do is find a nice boy and settle down. Grandpa can't for the life of him understand why you don't share his passion for World War Two memorabilia.

Just because they can't tell the difference between you and them doesn't mean you can't. They have their own (unconscious, unhealthy) reasons for not letting you step out into the world and be autonomous. The fact that they will be disappointed, angry, sad, or upset because you are is not your problem. It's theirs. If they can't let you go, you simply have to pry yourself away. I know that sounds harsh, but as some anonymous advice giver once said, "Children need roots to grow and wings to fly." So start flapping.

Of course, you and your folks both may enjoy or get something out of your dependence on them—they get gratification and you don't have to hurt their feelings and wise them up that you're an adult. Don't fret, you don't have to stop loving them, but you do have to start letting them know that you're going to exercise your rights as an adult however you see fit. This can be an excruciating process in some families. Remember, Mother or Father doesn't know best. You do!

▌ **GRAB YOUR THINKING CAP** Have you emotionally separated from your family? If not, why not, and what are you waiting for? ▌

Regulate intimacy

Intimacy means closeness. We all think we want it, but most of us are at least mildly ambivalent about it. What we want is the good part of it: companionship and that warm, fuzzy feeling of being loved, valued, and cared about. The bad parts we can do without: risk of abandonment and rejection or feeling smothered by too much of a good thing. The best any of us can do is to regulate intimacy. Relationships are never static; people move toward and away from each other emotionally as naturally as the tide rolls in and out. It's downright scary to want to be closer to a partner and be rebuffed because he or she has other things to do. It's equally bothersome when she or he wants to cozy up and the last thing you feel like doing is having a snuggle.

Regulating intimacy means enjoying both closeness and distance, basking in oneness as well as emotional breathing space. If you're like many people, you have trouble letting a partner know directly when you need space or closeness. You ask indirectly, drop hints, or desperately wish your partner would know what you want without your having to ask. Well, it's grown-up time, and grown-ups use words to tell other people how they feel and what they want: I'd love to spend time with you. I'd like a couple of hours to myself. Not now but maybe later. I want a hug. I'm too angry to talk right now. Could we cuddle?

If you haven't had terrific role models for regulating intimacy, you'll have a steep learning curve. Your tendency will be to do what your parents did or, in rebellion, the opposite. Regulation is a kind of inspired dance between you and another person. You can't do the steps well unless you can sense where your feet are; you can't regulate intimacy unless you know what's in your heart. It's essential to recognize what frightens you about closeness and distance and work through your issues, so that you know what you're feeling and can express it appropriately.

▐ **GRAB YOUR THINKING CAP** Fess up, why are you so terrified of getting too close or of having too much distance in intimate relationships? ▐

Value dependence and independence equally

Of all the difficult life skills all nice girls who are suffering from cookie jar–itis have to learn, the biggest is striking a balance between doing things yourself and getting help. You know it's true: You live to *give* help but get all squishy in the *seek*-help department. Do you understand why you insist on doing everything yourself (and then wonder why you're all stressed out)?

You have to answer this question in order to move into a healthy balance between the part of you that wishes to be independent and the part wishing to be dependent. *Is she crazy?* you're asking yourself. *Moi, wishing to be dependent?* Okay, Ms. Freud, here's a question I often ask clients, "Which is better, to be independent or dependent?" Usually they look at me like I just stepped out of a spaceship and quip, "Well, duh, independent, of course." Wrong (but the common) answer. I confess, it's a trick question because neither one is better than the other. Emotional health means knowing when to be independent and when to be dependent and valuing both equally. Simple as that. Now, please reread that sentence until it becomes tattooed on your brain.

We require the ability to be dependent *and* independent to live happily and successfully (and to steer clear of food when we're upset) because when we have problems, it often helps to turn to people. And to do so, we have to feel it's okay (not wrong, scary, or weak) to depend on them. We have to trust that they'll take us seriously, validate our feelings, and make every effort to help us feel better. Naturally, if your folks didn't regularly do this for you in childhood, you probably missed out on learning this skill.

The truth is, there are oodles of people out there who are trustworthy, caring, and supportive. They'd help you in a New York minute if you gave them half a chance. Of course, distinguishing them from self-centered, unempathic egoists wh should be avoided at all cost takes a while. The secret to discernment, once again, is staying connected to your feelings and not blinding yourself to reality. Trust comes from trial and error. You know, testing, testing, 1, 2, 3. You toss out an emotional crumb and see what someone does with it. Plus you pay mega-attention to overall patterns. On the whole, is someone there for you emotionally or does he or she change the subject when you share your feelings? Can you count on him or her to make you feel better, or do you come away from encounters feeling worse? If people are not up to the job of supporting you, then you have to consider the role you want them to play in your life, and I don't care whether we're talking about your mother, father, brother, sister, husband, boss, roommate, or alleged best friend.

Most nice girls pride themselves on their independence and are totally out of touch with their dependency needs (which everyone on the planet has)—except around food. You may hate having an eating jones but, let's face it, that's a lot less scary than needing people. Food sits still, people walk away. But if you want to stop with the food abuse, you need to learn how to trust and depend on (the right) people. Once you can take in more of what people have to give you, you'll feel fuller and more satisfied. Honest, people beat out food any day of the week! Establishing mutual interdependence, called simply give-and-take, will keep you in balance.

▮▮ **GRAB YOUR THINKING CAP** Why is it so hard for you to ask for help or take it when it's offered? Why is it okay to depend on food for solace but not people? ▮▮

Tolerate not being perfect
Ooo, is this a biggie. The topic is so huge that it gets its own chapter (see Chapter 8). For now, suffice it to say that learning

to tolerate your own imperfections will be one of your major tasks—and greatest hurdles. Accepting that you won't always be the best or do things right requires skill in a number of areas: allowing yourself to feel disappointment or shame and move on, learning from mistakes, tolerating regrets, taking calculated risks, bouncing back from failure, eliminating all-or-nothing thinking, learning to laugh at yourself, lowering expectations, and setting realistic goals. Tolerating imperfection means forgetting black and white, thinking in shades of gray, and assessing behavior in terms of gradients and continuums.

Self-regulate

Self-regulation is an art that involves knowing when enough is enough. It's described as a felt sense. What's a felt sense, you ask? An intuitive feeling, a gut reaction, a flash of insight that transmits information from you to you. Obviously, the word "enough" pops up a heck of a lot in the food arena when you ask yourself if you're hungry, full, or satisfied (you do ask yourself, don't you?). A sense of sufficiency can happen anytime, anyplace, over anything. You're using it when you say, I'm tired, bored with reading, tuckered out from running around, thirsty, hankering for company, itching to get away from the kids, peopled out, dying to be alone, or crazy to get out of the house.

When you trust your intuition and gut feelings, you look to them to help guide your life and keep it in balance. Nice girls have mega-difficulties with self-regulation: They give too much and take too little. Their valves are constantly open and they don't know how to shut them off. Or, more accurate, they see their valves only as on or off, not on low, medium low, medium high, or high. When you learn to regulate your caring for and about others, your me-o-stat will work better and you'll give more to yourself. When you get in touch with overdoing ar learn to self-regulate, you're more likely to return to neut rather than to stop doing completely (for example, instead of keeping away from the gym after going seven days a week, you'll settle on going three or four times weekly).

Learning to self-regulate takes time, practice, and patience. It can be frustrating because there's no right answer, and the process is more art than science. Only through trial and error will you learn. Become your own little science project. You may be tempted to ask someone else to set limits for you, but if you do, you'll never learn for yourself. The only way to develop a felt sense of what's enough is to buddy up with all your feelings (especially the yucky ones). When you improve at self-regulating, you'll notice a transformational change in your life and will be in greater harmony with yourself and the world around you.

❚ **GRAB YOUR THINKING CAP** In what situations do you get stuck in either the "on" or "off" position? ❚

Live purposefully as well as in the moment

Nice girls seem to swing in one of two directions. Either you're always making plans, living in the future, and missing out on today, or you're floating through life on automatic pilot doing what you're told, following what you learned in childhood, and spending your life trying to live up to unrealistic ideals and expectations—that half the time aren't even yours! Why bother getting up every day and busting your butt if you have no idea why you're doing what you're doing . . . and aren't even enjoying it? Are you a robot? If not, then you need to find your own purpose, passion, and meaning in life.

You may drift toward food because it's the most fun thing in your day. Do you get psyched about dining out because it's the most interesting and exciting part of your week? Adventures in food land do not a happy life make. Living purposely means setting realistic goals and then making conscious choices that move you toward them. And not living exclusively in or for the future. It's a tricky business staying in the moment while keeping aware of what lies ahead. When you're engaged in the moment and caught up in the positive momentum of life (called flow), you're too busy and happy to eat.

Generally, it's not the thinking about life that gets you, it's the emotions that knock you senseless. You agonize about what you *should* be doing, if you *need* to do better, if you *ought* to be doing something else. You worry and feel guilty and conflicted and don't get to enjoy every precious second. The truth is that staying connected to your feelings is exactly what helps you live a purposeful life because it tells you what makes you happy and what doesn't. If you tend toward anxiety and living in the future, you need to work on gently pushing it away and developing faith in your gut reactions. If you incline toward impulsivity and drifting mindlessly toward unforeseen consequences and vague life goals, you'll have to sit down and engage in a little heart-to-heart with yourself about the meaning of life in general and the meaning of yours in particular.

▮ **GRAB YOUR THINKING CAP** Quick, you have only one year to live. What will you do? ▮

There are other skills that enable you to create a good life, but by acquiring the eight above, you stand an excellent chance of shedding some of your niceness and inching up to the front of the line. Along the way, however, you'll have to pick up a complete kit of self-care strategies because if you're going to throw yourself into the thick of life, you need to be prepared for anything and everything. These strategies are the preventive and protective measures necessary to keep yourself in good working order—physically, mentally, and emotionally. You'll notice (I hope) that these behaviors and attitudes don't come from out of the blue but fall directly out of life care skills. Building the skills will make it easier to develop strategies, and practicing strategies will reinforce the skills.

Self-care strategies to learn

Say yes and no appropriately

This a high-wire act for everyone. The goal is to sense when you're in balance and when you're not and keep shifting slightly in one direction or another to regain equilibrium. Because life is constantly changing, you won't be able to stay in balance for long. Sometimes you'll feel as if you're doing too much and other times as if you're doing too little. That's natural and normal. The problem arises when you're stuck in a pattern of excess or insufficiency or ping-pong from one extreme to the other. By keeping in touch with your internal sufficiency meter and saying yes and no appropriately, you'll feel less overwhelmed and stressed, calmer and more centered. And, of course, less inclined to eat when you're not hungry.

Learn to delegate

This is the best strategy for reducing stress. No matter how energetic and talented you are, no woman is an island. Humans are designed for interchange and mutual dependence. Seeking help and delegating are ways you ensure that you don't overtax yourself (which often leads to unwanted eating). One of my most unfavorite words in the English language (or any other, for that matter) is "strong." We think we must be strong; we strive to be strong. Workhorses need to be strong, but people should be flexible. Healthy means knowing when you can do something yourself and when you can't. It involves changing your mind if you made the wrong decision and reveling in the fact that people can and will help you.

Avoid triangulation

This is probably a new strategy for you. You may not even know what it means. Triangulation refers to any kind of interpersonal triangle—think of it as not getting caught in the middle of two (or more) people's craziness. When you try to smooth over a blowout between your mother and sister that doesn't involve you, you're getting triangulated. The same is true when your daughter and husband or two best friends are battling, or two bigwigs at work are in conflict. If it has nothing to do with you, reduce your stress, step back, and uncomfortable as that makes you, stop trying to fix the problem and stay out of it!

Balance social and alone time

This is a favorite topic in women's magazines. There's no magic way of making time other than carving it out and sticking to your guns. I don't care if you sit in the middle of your living room floor naked staring at your chipped nails. Most people who have trouble being alone are so anxious when there aren't people around or when they're not busy, that they freak (and turn to food). That's because when you're alone, you start to experience your true feelings: confusion, anger, loneliness, depression, anxiety. These emotions have value. You may not know what to do when you're alone other than think about what you should do. Spend enough time by yourself and something will surface. Cross my heart.

Balance work and play

Reaching a balance encourages you to throw yourself into goal-oriented tasks and feel good about accomplishments (which adds to a sense of competence and builds self-esteem) *and* allows you to turn off your motor and recharge your battery. No one can run on empty! Play and relaxation are not wrong or due to laziness or lack of motivation. They are natural and normal. If your motor is constantly running, what is it running from? Perhaps it's your idealized view of yourself, what someone else would (or does) say about the evils of idle hands. An addiction to work, overscheduling, and busyness are unhealthy and add to stress. Balancing work and play gives you the best of both worlds.

Handle emotions

If you can do this well, you will reduce stress considerably. As described under life skills, there are three components to emotional management: experiencing and tolerating uncomfortable/painful emotions, expressing feelings appropriately and effectively, and containing and soothing feelings. Even though it may feel totally debilitating at first to sit with distressing feelings, you're really taking utmost care of yourself because you're learning what's going on inside you. Building emotional muscle takes time and practice, but even trying it out will keep you away from the refrigerator.

Expressing feelings helps you blow off steam whether you're having a good cry by yourself, venting to a friend, or telling someone exactly how he or she hurt you. Containing and soothing emotions involves positive self-talk, self-compassion, distracting yourself from pain rather than dwelling on it, and finding ways to relax. Most nice girls sit on feelings until they explode, a very poor self-care strategy indeed. First, stress builds to the breaking point, then shame follows an outburst. Take care of your emotions and they'll take care of you!

Tolerate other people's emotions

Hurting people and allowing them to feel bad is a special skill subset in handling emotions. We can't avoid hurting people's feelings. The best we can do is to be aware when we do and try (at least initially) to do it as gently as possible. The rule of thumb is as follows: *It's okay to hurt another person's feelings if you are doing it in the service of taking care of yourself.* Therefore, if someone is disappointed because you can't do something for him, so be it. If someone is hurt because you're not who she would like you to be, tough toddies. Life isn't fair, for you, me, or anyone else and we all must learn how to get over unintentionally hurt feelings.

Another aspect of this issue is allowing people to feel bad no matter what the cause: Loved ones die and we grieve, we don't get all the things we want in life (kids, fame, jobs, life partners, the Nobel Prize), people come and go in our lives, love doesn't last, etc. You take care of yourself when you let people experience their feelings. It's not your job to put a Band-Aid on every boo-boo (except with children and, even then, children need to learn how to manage disappointment and hurt). Every adult has to learn how to take care of his or her own feelings. Another rule of thumb: If somebody has to hurt, please let it not be you.

Minimize/avoid contact with toxic people

This is tough but essential to self-care. Here's a bulletin that may astound you: You are not obligated to be around anyone who is regularly not as nice to you as you are to him or her. That includes folks who invalidate, belittle, and ignore your feelings, are purposefully hurtful, don't care how you feel, and are neglectful or abusive. I don't care who these people are, you want to stay as far away from them as possible. Stop feeling sorry for them and realize that they push people away and it's their own fault. Obviously, you can't always avoid certain people—a boss, parent, relative, or neighbor. But you don't have to court their company either. Limit contact with people who detract from your life, whether they like it or not.

Focus energy on fixing you, not others

What a sticky wicket—but it's at the core of effective self-care. It's a lot easier to throw your energy into fixing another broken person than to mend yourself, but it's a thankless, draining job that is essentially unproductive and self-destructive. I adore being a therapist, but I get paid for taking care of others! It's obviously necessary to take good care of children and anyone with severe physical infirmities or without working mental faculties, but keep away from stubborn, manipulative know-it-alls who only want to hook you into their lives and have no intention of changing. These victims will suck the life out of you and you'll end up recharging yourself with food. You are responsible only for yourself! Isn't that enough?

Enjoy praise, take credit, and have good feelings

This is something one would think you'd want to do automatically. Unfortunately, you are much better at believing that you haven't done enough (and feeling guilt, shame, etc.) than believing that you've done a super job and feeling happy about it. Nice girls are terrible at taking compliments and credit. They're full of "aw gosh" and "who, me?" Believe it or not, accepting praise is part of good self-care. You're not going to get a swelled head merely because you enjoy a "thank you" for a job well done; you're not going to become a braggart because you crow a bit. It's not an attractive quality for you always to be putting yourself down. More than that, you need to glory in the glorious feelings so you can handle the times you don't get or deserve them. At the risk of sounding redundant, it's good to have good feelings.

Learn to take criticism and feedback without personalizing

What a doozy of a skill for any of us. It's never fun to hear negative things about yourself. However, it needn't be a knife in the back either. Listen up, you're going to do some things well and some things poorly just like the rest of us schmoes. Not every criticism is meant to rip your heart out. Not every insult or piece of criticism is true. The best advice is to remember this adage: If it comes out of someone else's mouth—even if it has your name attached to it—the sentiment belongs to him or her. It's that person's thoughts and feelings, not yours. Of course, you don't want to tune out all feedback. Self-care means hearing everyone out, then making up your mind *yourself* whether what is said has validity and value. If so, swell, learn from it. If not, delete it.

Take good care physically and mentally

This means developing strategies to keep your mind active and challenged and your body healthy. It includes everything from getting medical checkups to wearing weather-appropriate clothing to finding passion in life. No surprise, but a nice girl is likely to cancel a mammogram to drive a friend to hers. If you don't value and take care of your body, it's going to fall apart, and then where will you be? You'll *really* be dependent on others—one of your worst nightmares. Good self-care (from eating to exercise to rest) is one of the easier ways to start putting yourself first. Make a doctor's appointment you've postponed, buy a new dress or pair of shoes, have your hair cut attractively, take vitamins, get some sleep, buy a novel by your favorite author. Mental self-care means getting out of ruts and

...ines, thinking out of the box, and challenging your brain. You are precious (in spite of your overniceness—or maybe even because of it), so let yourself sparkle.

Did you notice that not one life skill or self-care strategy involved food? In fact, I could have gone on for another ten pages and never mentioned eating. Building life skills and developing self-care strategies involve every fiber of your being, every part of you—except your appetite. A cookie once in a blue moon or a night out on the town at some fabulous, expensive restaurant when you're feeling especially blue is fine, but self-care means having a host of tricks up your sleeve, not a brownie.

▮ GRAB YOUR THINKING CAP How would you take care of yourself if there was no such thing as food on earth? ▮

So now you know what you have to do to give up food as a best friend and, corny as it sounds, become your own best buddy—a self-advocate who knows when to be nice and when to be naughty, who gets a kick out of pleasing other people but gets a bigger kick out of making nice to herself, who can say yes and no in the right balance, who loves herself better than anyone, and treats herself that way!

NICE GIRL RECOVERY TIPS

- Assess which life skills you've got a pretty good handle on and which ones you're clueless about. Make a plan for improvement that includes asking for lots of help. Don't feel you must change overnight or give up all the wonderful qualities you love about yourself—your kindheartedness, generosity, compassion for the underdog—but think about adding traits to your personality.

- Assess your self-care skills and how well they work. If you don't have enough self-care strategies to keep you afloat, brainstorm new ones and try them out. Give each one at least a three-week trial. Make sure to include strategies that both foster strengthening your emotional resources and reaching out to other people.

- Have a serious conversation with yourself about emotional eating and what you can do about it. Pick one or two self-care strategies to start using immediately to avoid abusing food.

To do today

Be honest with how you feel toward someone rather than lying to him or her and yourself.

Meet One of the Nice Girls

Carol now

Carol is a sixty-one-year-old former policewoman, one year into retirement. Her specialty is dealing with sexual abuse victims and she has won numerous citations from the city for the work she has done on and off the job. She enters treatment with me because she can't get used to not working full-time. Part of her is relieved to be rid of the perpetual stress and pressure her very difficult job entailed, and the other part longs for her adrenaline-filled days. She admits that, like many people in her field, she had become addicted to the constant need for her services and the rush of being on the go nearly every minute.

A widow of five years, Carol is trying to make a life for herself but says she was just getting used to living without her husband when she "had to learn to cope with retirement." All the free time on her hands makes her jittery and uneasy and so she has taken a couple of volunteer jobs, mostly helping rape and sexual abuse survivors. She and her husband had no children together, although he had a son from a previous, short-lived marriage who lived with them part-time growing up. The couple enjoyed a busy lifestyle, especially camping, biking, and hiking together—the outdoors was their salvation.

Carol refuses to admit she has eating problems but holds herself on a very short leash around food. She weighs herself daily and counts calories and fat grams. She was a fat child who was teased unmercifully and says she'll "never, ever put myself in that position again." Because of all her free time, she goes to the gym daily and can spend as much as three hours working out. If she has an especially long or arduous workout, she allows herself an ice cream cone or piece of chocolate cake. She says that counting calories doesn't bother her a bit and, in fact, brings her satisfaction. She likes being in control of her eating and weight, and is convinced that being a bit overzealous is a small price to pay to stay in shape.

Most of the time when I ask Carol what she's feeling, she is unsure, remarking that, other than stress, she's never thought much about emotions. Feelings weren't something that she shared with her husband or anyone, even friends. When I do my spiel on the nature and purpose of emotions, it's as if I'm speaking a foreign tongue. The only reason she knows she's anxious, she admits, is that her primary care doctor told her she needed to manage her anxiety better to control her blood pressure.

Carol as a child

No surprise that she's the daughter of a policeman—actually, of two policemen. Her father died when she was a toddler and her mother, a probation officer, remarried her stepfather shortly after. Carol has two brothers, both in the military overseas, with whom she's always been close. She was highly competitive with them and always wished she'd been born a boy. In Carol's family, everyone did what he or she was told with minimal fuss. As she puts it, "We learned to take orders real early." She can't remember ever seeing her mother, father, or stepfather cry or exhibit any emotion other than anger or frustration. "If they did, I never saw it."

Carol was raped by a classmate at the police academy. He was expelled and she went through a terrible time with everyone knowing what had happened and being solicitous of her. She declined prosecuting her rapist, however, because she only wanted the incident to go away. Although she was sent to counseling, she couldn't figure out what she was supposed to talk about and just showed up every week until she was discharged. Other than the academy therapist, she's never talked to anyone about the rape until our sessions—not her parents, brothers, or husband. It was simply something that happened and was best put behind her.

De-nicing Carol

Although you might not envision Carol as our typical nice girl, she's a good girl at heart: She doesn't want to burden other people with her feelings, follows orders, and throws herself into taking care of others, especially victims. Nor is she an overeater like most of the nice women in this book. However, the vigilance she exerts over her eating and body smacks of regimentation and restriction and indicates how much she fears losing control and becoming fat once more. As are many nice girls, she is driven by shame.

It takes a long while for Carol to recognize how disconnected she is from her emotional self and how she uses keeping busy and controlling her weight to distract from her emotions. Much of our work is revisiting her childhood, with me fishing for feelings and her swimming away. She isn't sure what she might find, but whatever it is, she fears it will destroy her image of herself as the good daughter, policewoman, wife, and stepmother. I'm usually one step ahead of clients, but regarding her childhood, I'm not exactly sure what she might discover either. Is there repressed abuse by her mother, father, stepfather, or brothers? Did something happen before the rape to make her become sealed over? We don't know yet and may never know.

We have better luck talking about the rape, and Carol is positively shocked to uncover layers of emotions she never dreamed she had. She's now less fearful of her intense emotions than amazed she's had them all along and buried them. Of course, once we start picking at the rape, off come the scabs over the loss of her husband and the ending of her career, and out pours the grief. It's tough going for her, but there's also something that Carol finds cathartic in letting it all hang out—the anger at her husband for dying prematurely before they could enjoy retirement together, rage over the rape, and all the mixed emotions over her career. My validating her emotions brings her enormous relief.

We can't talk about her control issues without exploring her history as a fat child who was teased and shamed, and her current rigid approach to eating and maintaining her weight. After some time, Carol starts to experiment with not counting calories, but it's too anxiety producing and she resumes the practice. She agrees to try the experiment again sometime in the future but for now is holding on to what works for her.

What's Next? *In Chapter 4, "Taking Care of Family,"*
you'll learn

- How your brain gets "pruned" to encourage and discourage specific personality traits

- The effect of parental role models and family interactions on how nice you become

- How to stop being overinvolved with your family of origin

FOUR

I Am Woman, Hear Me Chew!

Taking Care of Family

Ah, the family. Little ones nestled in their beds, progeny making us proud, siblings there for each other, parents with open arms offering practical wisdom, grandparents thriving in their golden years. Not your family snapshot? Not living a series of Hallmark moments? Well, join the club, because neither is anyone else.

Erma Bombeck wrote a book with a brilliant title that says it all: *Family—The Ties That Bind . . . and Gag!* Whether we're talking family of origin (our parents) or procreation (our children), like most things, the *f* word is a mixed bag (often of nuts!). Some of the best moments of our lives occur with family and, sadly, so do some of our worst. Even if we move far away from parents and relatives, even after all of them are dead and buried, they are still with us—in our hearts, our memories, and the myriad ways that knowing them has shaped our lives for better or worse.

When we're children, most of us believe our problems with parents and siblings will end when we grow up, when we're all equals. Ha! We merely have more devious and perilous ways of trying to feel better when we find ourselves starring in our own version of *Family Feud*. Now, I'm not saying that we don't have choices as adults that we didn't have as children, or that we shouldn't hope to act more maturely around family than we did when we were, say, seven. I am saying that difficulties with our first group experience will continue to plague us unless we get a firm handle on them.

Sure, some people have a fabulous, genuinely close, meaningful relationship with their kin—differences are accepted, no one tries to control or manipulate anyone else, each member has a say and is valued for his or her uniqueness, disagreements are settled sensibly with no hard feelings, and everyone works hard to make sure he or she contributes to keeping the family a loving unit. However, families like this are few and far between compared to the ones that roil your stomach and break your heart. Most of us have major and minor long-standing grievances against our parents, siblings, and other relatives even as we love and care deeply about them. So we limp along, managing the best we know how, which is usually how we managed as kids—keeping quiet, escaping, tuning out, trying too hard to please, eating when we're upset—without reflecting on why we act the way we do or how we act differently.

Those of you who are dues-paying members of the over-nice club are especially at risk for falling into family traps that stress you to the max and make you want to seek solace in your cupboard. But if you don't attend to your own needs around family, you put yourself in great jeopardy for using food for all the wrong reasons. This is true whether we're talking about your family of origin or of creation. To grow healthier, as well as to develop a positive relationship with food, you need to reflect on exactly where being so darned nice with your family has gotten you. You also have to understand why you've chosen to put family ahead of yourself.

Don't we all want to be nice to our family?

There's a difference between being nice to family and being able to click off the nice channel when necessary. Being kind, generous, and giving are splendid qualities, but employing them exclusively and not tapping into other personality traits around family is unhealthy and not in your self-interest. The goal is not to be un-nice but to make sure you use all the cards in your personality deck.

Let's take a look at niceness—a word reeking of goodness, politeness, and rule following—and the family. Most parents probably think they're nice to their children and encourage their children to be nice to them. When a teacher or neighbor says, "Trish is such a nice little girl," Mommy and Daddy beam with pride and believe they're model parents. Remember, "nice" is a catchall word referring to anything from a first grader thanking her teacher for after-school help to a child sitting quietly in her seat not daring to challenge a teacher who yells constantly and runs the classroom like a platoon. Nice easily translates into not being a pain in the butt, which is how too many adults wish kids to be.

While most children do want to be nice to family members, its importance runs along a continuum based on family priorities. If niceness (appropriate behavior, caring, giving, etc.) is prized above all else, children usually catch on and strive in that direction. Equally, if intelligence is highly esteemed, boys and girls try to outdo each other in the smart department and bring home all A's. The same can be said for being musical, athletic, popular, community minded, and almost any trait you can think of because the almost singular underlying (and unconscious) objective of children is to obtain parental love and approval.

Do I have too much "nice wiring" in my head?

Kinda. Here's how it happens. We start off as tiny infant approval seekers to get fed and cared for. As we mature and are able to make choices, in basic Pavlovian response—punishment for "bad" behavior and reward for "good"—we act in very specific ways to get our emotional and physical needs met, not because we're filled with some lofty, higher purpose, but to survive and flourish. In healthy families, children learn by consistently getting rewarded for healthy behavior and by being fairly punished when they behave poorly. Like flowers and plants that grow toward the sun, we automatically grow toward love. As youngsters, we'll do and put up with almost anything for that internal glow that comes from positive attention and praise, that nearly indescribable feeling that's like warm syrup running through our veins and makes us smile and smile.

The directions in which we grow are determined by the traits genetically passed down to us through our DNA (nature) and the behaviors that get reinforced (nurture)—or not. We develop unique personalities through a fascinating process in the brain called "pruning." The brain is an amazingly flexible organ. The plasticity, or malleability, of the brain enables us to learn behavior, as well as unlearn it and learn new behavior. The brain's ability to change through learning is called neuroplasticity.

Exactly how does the brain change? Pruning is an automatic activity that is similar to how you shape a rosebush or a hedge. Our infant brains are programmed to develop nerve cells that process the flood of sensory information being received. A basic "trunk line" gets established and cells branch out and make connections with one another in a form of communication. During development, connections that are not reinforced die out, while ones that are reinforced get strengthened. Repeated experience encourages neurological pathways to grow, so that connections that are activated the most are the ones that stick around. Your particular experience (along with your DNA) determines your unique set of neural connections.

Are you getting the picture? When you receive parental approval in the form of hearing "good girl" for letting your younger brother play with your train set (even though he broke the last two cabooses), your brain is being molded (for better or worse) toward niceness. The same thing happens when you're encouraged not to throw your popcorn into the hair of the person in front of you at the movies and when you receive a lollipop for not crying in the checkout line in the supermarket. This pruning is necessary so that you'll fit into society, but how the brain gets shaped also depends on what aspects of personality your parents value. Do most Moms and Dads strongly value Little Lucy questioning authority, rebelling, thinking for herself, and being outspoken? Yeah, right. Most (but, thankfully, not all) parents want their children to be well behaved because it makes parental lives easier, and also because they believe it will bring their children happiness and success in society.

For women especially, those values too often include fitting in, keeping quiet, not making waves, ministering to others, and putting ourselves last. So one reason we end up pursuing niceness as we mature is that our brains have been pruned in that direction. Impulses to speak up, challenge others, take risks, be selfish, focus on our own needs, and make our own way are discouraged by family and culture, and eventually those neural pathways die out. At the same time, neural pathways that make us considerate, other-oriented caretakers are getting stoked to the max and are, therefore, growing by leaps and bounds. With all the nudging women get in the direction of sainthood, it's a wonder our heads aren't lopsided!

So now you know how, on the most basic, physiological level, you learn to be nice at the hands of your family and why it's so hard to undo the damage. Change means nothing short of snipping off your "nice" neural connections and making sure that other ones get plenty of fertilizer and reinforcement. The chance of that happening when you're a child is slim to none. You don't have much say in your life and are beholden to grown-ups every step of the way. Unless outside forces are strong and constant, you're stuck in the hands of the people with the pruning shears—your family. For the most part, at least until you reach adolescence, they are the pruners and you are the prunee.

Pruning happens in two ways. One is how you're treated, that is, the interactions you have with your early caretakers. The other is what you observe, or the role modeling they consciously or unconsciously display. Therefore, some of your brain shaping happens consciously when Mom says, "Jenny, stop pestering Daddy while he's watching football. Be a good girl and go play with your Hannah Montana doll." A more unconscious molding occurs when Dad snaps at Mom for interrupting him with an important question while he's watching a golf match and she retreats in guilty silence. The message is that Mom needs to put Dad's feelings above her own.

So when you're considering how you got to be as nice as you are to your family and everyone else (you *are* thinking about it, aren't you?), you have to examine both what you were told and what you observed. Too often, when trying to figure out what makes us tick, we focus only on what our parents said and did to us, what was obvious or, in psych language, on *manifest* messages we received. What's often far more telling are the *latent* messages that came from what parents said to and did with each other. I like to picture children as adorable, brightly colored little sponges with huge eyes and big antennae—all the better to see, hear, and pick up on everything that happens around them. The manifest messages we can usually deal with; it's the latent ones that are the doozies, secretly feeding us information about how to think and behave when we have no idea our brains are even open for business.

▌ **GRAB YOUR THINKING CAP** What role modeling went on in your family that encouraged females to be nice and discouraged them from being anything else? ▌

How does all this brain stuff relate to how I treat my family?

We develop our attitudes toward family according to templates laid down through brain pruning in childhood. If your template has your mother and other female relatives putting aside their needs to serve your family, it's natural that you will end up trying to walk in their shoes. Monkey see, monkey do. Not only do you learn to be nice, you also learn that there are certain very specific ways to act as a female. There's a script you must follow and prescribed roles you must play. Or else!

For example, who had the power in your family? I don't mean who got to decide what shade of beige the bedroom drapes would be or whether your gym shorts were dirty enough to go into the laundry. Who made the major decisions and had the final say most of the time? Who controlled the money, including where you went on vacation and what big-ticket items the family purchased? Who retreated first during an argument, tried to smooth over problems, bent over backward to keep the peace, was considered the family worrywort?

In the traditional family, Dad leads and Mom (and kiddies) follow. Yes, customs are slowly changing—though on average women earn only 77 percent of what men are paid for the same work.[2] Of course, if you were raised by a single mom (with or without help from others), you know that women can be feisty and capable. Single moms—single dads, too—have to do it all. Plus many of you may have had stepmoms and stepdads who were far different from your birth parents. You may have seen one dynamic with one set of parents and quite a different set with another. Moreover, family interactions can change over time. Rare is the relationship that remains completely static over the years, but there are some in which spouses confine themselves to rigid roles out of which they never stray. What you're looking to identify is the general tenor of who took care of what and whom.

If both parents were around, think about who had the power in the relationship and in the family and who did the emotional caretaking. In some families, it's painfully obvious: Father never lifts a finger except to click the remote or point blame, while Mother runs herself ragged trying to be Wonder Woman. Or Dad has a drinking problem and Mom must keep the family peace and the family from going to pieces. Of course, there are families in which the scenario is reversed: Mom is chronically depressed and Dad works, tends to her needs, and is the chief emotional caretaker as well. However, generally it's the woman taking care of the man and kids.

■ GRAB YOUR THINKING CAP Growing up in your family, which parent

- made the big decisions?
- did the emotional caretaking?
- made the most or greatest sacrifices?
- was the people pleaser?
- had to have the final word?
- frightened you or your siblings the most?
- made sure his or her own needs were met?
- backed off from getting his or her own needs met?
- enabled the other by covering for or minimizing his or her personal or professional inadequacies?
- caused most of the problems and didn't much care?
- was the worrier and emotional problem solver?
- held the family together? **■**

In our society, men tend to take care of things and women tend to take care of people. I've also heard a similar sentiment: Men see objects and women see the relationships between objects. Some of this perspective is assuredly hardwired, but the rest is due to plain old repetition throughout social and family history—one generation teaches the next, which teaches the next, and so on and so forth.

In my experience, women who grow up overly nice have commonalities in their upbringing regarding caretaking based on gender-based templates. Here are some common ones.

Mother did it all

In this family type, Mother was a human dynamo, an amazing powerhouse who worked, kept house, and took care of the children, all with an eye to perfection. She was the ultimate service provider. She'd cancel a dental appointment for her toothache to whisk you to dance class or break a movie date with a girlfriend to stay home with Dad who was in a funk and "needed" company. She ran from fire to fire, putting out flames and never seemed to rest. If she wasn't scrubbing the floor, she was teaching you how to roller-skate or learning how to make the tapioca pudding recipe you had at your friend's house. She hosted most family holiday dinners and insisted on making everything herself—from scratch. The woman excelled at almost everything and always strived to get things right, yet had a hard time taking compliments and giving herself credit. From her you learned that a woman must do everything perfectly, not to seek out or accept credit or praise, to put other people's wishes before yours, and that doing good for others is more acceptable than doing good for yourself. Like Mom, you jump in to solve problems and crises but never feel you're doing enough.

Mother's main job was taking care of Father

In some unfortunate families, Dad had physical, mental, or emotional problems and couldn't function adequately as a spouse or parent. Maybe he was irresponsible and got fired from job after job. Maybe he was a gambler or spent money like water so that the family lived on a shoestring budget with the wolf howling at the door. Perhaps he was a blowhard, liar, and cheat with a raging temper who repeatedly embarrassed the family. He might have been so depressed that he often threatened suicide, requiring Mom constantly to bolster his fragile ego so he didn't bottom out. In my experience, a substantial number of nicer-than-nice women had fathers who were alcoholic, leading them to bouts of rage, binges in which they disappeared for days, lose good jobs, erratic behavior (flying high one minute and crashing the next or alternating complete disinterest in the family with overindulgence and over-the-top concern or demands), associations with unsavory characters, excessive self-pity, diminished accountability, and blame others (like the ever-so-convenient Mom and the kids) for all their problems.

Worse, many markedly nice women had fathers who abused them and their mothers, physically or emotionally (and sometimes sexually). These women were either victims of abuse or watched as Dad knocked around Mom or their siblings. Many of these women may consider Mom a heroine rather than a victim who was unable or unwilling to take herself and kids out of harm's way. The template in this dynamic is simple and straightforward: other first, self last, no matter what. These wives and mothers did the best they could—for that matter, so did the errant fathers—in spite of the fact that their best clearly failed to be good enough. Occasionally roles were reversed and Dad put up with it all while Mom was the family antagonist. If you identified strongly with him, and many young girls do, you grow up with the same faulty ideas about relationships and the same fixed set of unhelpful values.

Mother was narcissistic and didn't really give a hoot about the family

Often nice girls are products of mothers who put themselves above everyone else in the family. Mom would leave the kids home with inappropriate babysitters to go out with her girl-friends while Dad was working overtime. Or she'd buy expensive clothes for herself while her children went to school in dirty hand-me-downs. Some of these mothers had mental problems—often untreated bipolar disorder, which causes marked mood swings—on top of being self-centered, and their children didn't know what to expect from one moment to the next.

If you grew up with a mom like this, all you may have wished for and dreamed of was a mother who did maternal things like bake cookies, buy you nice dresses, and take you to the park like friends' mothers did. As an adult, you may want to be as different from your mother as you possibly can be: Whereas she thought only of herself, you think only of others; whereas she regularly put herself first, you put yourself last; whereas she fussed nonstop over herself, you have a hard time doing anything kind for little old you. Well, you get the picture. You're so afraid of turning into your mother that you run in the opposite direction.

Mom and Dad were both poor caretakers

Sometimes both parents work and the oldest or most competent child is stuck at home being the parental surrogate or parentified child. She—yes, it's usually a she, even if there's an older boy— does the cooking, cleaning, and mothering of younger children on top of going to school. Often, parentified kids get praised for doing scut work and are punished when younger siblings in their care misbehave. Is that crazy-making, or what?

It's easy to see how an overburdened little girl would grow up to be a woman who is not only terrific at caretaking but also *knows no other way of relating to people.* Taking care of others is what got her the smidgen of approval she received, and she's afraid people will be angry with her if she fails to do it. The truth is she's clueless about what it's like to let other people take care of her because she's missed out on that formative experience. Now she's so used to being in charge and in control that, even though she may hate it, she can't give it up. What a crummy dilemma when someone wants to do things for her: Should she risk having someone take care of her? What if she likes it and wants it to continue? What if that person changes his or her mind and stops?

A child has to take care of her parents

In the all-time worst role reversal possible, some children have to take care of their parents in order to survive. If the parents have mental illness or substance abuse problems, these grow-up-too-fast progeny end up doing things like dragging a depressed mom out of bed, forcing her to eat breakfast, and pushing her out the door to get to work on time; paying bills because Dad is too irresponsible to be left with such a critical task; or calling Dad's boss and inventing stories about why he can't make it to the office when he's sleeping it off on the couch.

Rarely do overly responsible children enjoy even the approval that children who take care of their siblings get because Mom and Dad are too self-absorbed, needy, busy, depressed, or ashamed to recognize the exceptional job they're doing. These children never have a real childhood and caretaking is all they know: Life is a constant battle to juggle responsibilities and stay on top of things. It always feels as if they're not doing enough because there's so much to do. They can't ask for help because there's no one to give it and can't stop doing what they do because they fear their family and world will fall apart. Either way, not doing it all themselves is too frightening to contemplate and makes them feel like a failure. They're caught in a vise with no way out.

So if I'm stuck being a caretaker, why shouldn't I go commune with a doughnut?

Whoa, not so fast. Just because you learned to be a star caretaker doesn't mean you're branded for life. Now is a good time to step back and consider just how much you've fallen into the super-doer of family relations. Some of what you do may be fine; caretaking in itself is a good thing, a very good thing. As with food, however, you don't want to go overboard. Take a minute to review your role in your family of origin and also consider how you act with family now.

- Do family members gape in amazement at all you do, while you secretly feel you're not doing enough?

- Do you have health problems because you're exhausted and overweight?

- Are you an enabler for a spouse, child, sibling, or parent?

- Do you allow family members to take care of you and enjoy their ministrations?

- Are you the person relatives always call when they need something?

- Does the rest of your family pull its weight in age-, skill-, financial-, and time-appropriate ways?

- Do you get sucked into family squabbles rather than allow members to settle differences themselves?

- Must you host every family gathering (by choice or due to family pressure)?

- Are you afraid that if you stop doing all you do for the family either one member or the whole family will fall apart?

- Do you give your all because you can't stand saying no, living with guilt, having family members angry at or disappointed in you, or feeling selfish?

- Does your power in the family come from making members beholden to you because you do so much for them?

- Does the word "yes" pop out of your mouth automatically in response to family requests and cause you to be overburdened and overwhelmed?

Well, *that* should give you a good idea of whether you're just an average caretaker or going for the gold. Please, please, please don't judge yourself, but do try to see yourself honestly and accept that this is where you're at right now. Remember the old plastic brain and why you're reading this book. You're going to learn how to change and relate to family in different, healthier ways. It's not going to be easy and it won't be fun, but your current life is no picnic either. Odds are you won't change your nature and you don't have to worry about becoming selfish (a huge secret fear of nice women). You'll slam on the breaks long before you ever come anywhere near selfish!

Family members are difficult to manage whether they come from your loins or you come from theirs. If they're an ongoing energy drain, consider that interactions may not be healthy. Sure, sometimes there's a crisis and you have to run yourself ragged for a short period of time because of it: Your son breaks his leg the day after your mother goes into the hospital for a heart transplant and your dog just gave birth to the largest litter of puppies on record. This qualifies as a crisis and you will undoubtedly rise to the occasion. But crises by definition are temporary. Your elderly dad adamantly refusing to get help mowing the lawn or your teenage daughter demanding that you drive her over to her friend's house every day when the bus stop is around the corner are not crises. They are ongoing situations that need to be managed differently.

I'd be remiss if I didn't mention family situations in which you're not looking to be a superhero but are put in the position of miracle worker against your will: Your child is badly injured or has serious, chronic health problems and needs extra ongoing attention, Mom had a stroke six months after Dad's heart attack and they don't have the money for much outside care, or you're a single mom with a demanding job attending night school to better yourself. In these situations, you know that your life is going to be hectic and taxing for a very long time. What can you do but rise to the occasion? Even in these circumstances, however, there are women who make sure to continue taking care of themselves well while others let themselves go.

❚ GRAB YOUR THINKING CAP How much do you overdo with family? Do you prevent family members from being responsible for themselves or growing up? What do you get out of your Superwoman role? ❚❚

What is it about being with family that makes me crazy . . . and hungry?

Not surprising, if anyone can push your buttons, family members can. After all, they not only know what all your buttons are, some of them were responsible for creating them to begin with. One of the biggest problems with food and family is that they're both around a lot—together. You're visiting your mother, sitting in her kitchen drinking coffee surrounded by food, out with your sister for a monthly dinner, making lunch or a snack for the kids at home. When family comes to visit, it's often for a meal, especially a holiday one.

Another reason family interactions can make you nutty is that family history goes back such a long way. Within your family of origin, you've been playing nice girl for decades. You're locked into particular ways of relating that you and they are probably not even aware of. They can shoot up your blood pressure by a look or a word and make you want to beat a fast retreat before you've even taken off your coat.

Moreover, we like to put family in a special, idealized category—the people who have to take us in, the folks who will go to any lengths for us because we're blood, those who love us most (or so they say). We often expect more from family than from nonfamily members, which makes it even worse when they let us down. We might let other folks get away with being ignorant or petty or having faults in general, but we have high standards for relatives, just as they do for us. Especially if you're the Jill-of-all-trades and family caretaker, the assumptions and expectations members have of you is a setup for high stress and low satisfaction all around. And for you climbing into your kitchen cabinet and staying there.

Okay, okay already, you might be saying, *I get it. Sometimes I'm more there for family members than for myself, but what can I do about it in practical terms? I just can't stop being me and turn into someone else overnight. I have responsibilities and I'm not gonna drop 'em all and fly off to Tahiti tomorrow with Brad Pitt!* Of course you're not. Far be it from me to suggest that you go from being a goody-goody to a good-for-nothing. To give you a taste of what to do in real, practical, everyday terms, I've developed a No More Nice Girl Manifesto for you to live by around your family, a list of dos and don'ts for how to think and behave to give yourself that nice-ectomy you need and start turning around your relationship with food.

NO MORE NICE GIRL MANIFESTO FOR FAMILY

DO

• Maintain lots of contact with family members who are kind and caring about you and avoid ones who are energy drainers and aren't looking out for your interests.

• Make sure that family members are doing their fair share (in physical, financial, and emotional terms) to make the family unit work.

• Prioritize attending family events and get-togethers rather than attend them all and feel resentful or not go and feel guilty.

• Ask for help taking care of difficult family members (poor old Aunt Kathy who complains about everything to everyone) or ones whose care is time-consuming (your wheelchair-bound son with muscular dystrophy).

• Seek balance in relationships. If you're taking physical care of someone who can't do for himself, he should at the very least be appreciative and thank you in every way he can.

• Take time for yourself whether family members like it or not.

• Tell family members when they are too demanding and their requests are out of line.

• Teach your children to come to you when they truly need help (physical or emotional) and to work things out for themselves when they're able.

• Opt out of any adult living arrangement that is not mutual and where you feel like someone's mother or maid. Others need to grow up and you need to let them.

• Delegate tasks even if family members don't do things as well or as quickly as you'd like. You've been aspiring to be superhuman all your life. Give them a chance to learn how to be responsible for themselves.

- Develop and maintain close relationships with people outside the family. The experience will be refreshing and give you a new perspective on your blood ties.

DON'T

- Feel sorry for family members who are such miserable characters that they've pushed everyone else away. They made their bed, so (except in life-or-death situations) let them lie in it.

- Believe that you're indispensable. You'd like to think so and perhaps family members would too, but you're not. No one is.

- Let any family member guilt-trip you into doing anything you don't want to.

- Feel you have to do everything yourself and that you're weak if you ask for help.

- Automatically say yes to family requests. Instead, get into the habit of saying, "Let me think about it and get back to you."

- Infantilize family members whether they're old or young. Don't prevent them from doing what they're capable of and what is age appropriate.

- Be a poor role model for your children by not taking care of yourself. If you insist on being one, make sure this book stays in good condition 'cause they're gonna need it.

- Try to be strong all the time. Instead, aim for mentally healthy, which is a combination of independent, dependent, and interdependent.

- Let family members undermine your self-esteem, self-worth, or self-care—ever.

- Allow family members to tell you that you're a selfish you-know-what just because you want to take time for yourself. Most likely they're the selfish ones.

- Play peacemaker in family squabbles. The role of mediator is stressful and you don't want to go from peacemaker to pacemaker.

Well, now that you've had your first lesson in self-care, how does it feel? Terrifying, exhilarating, overwhelming, a bit of all three? Pay attention to whether you're thinking about food to take away uncomfortable feelings. Instead of wending your way toward the kitchen, just experience your emotions and reflect on what you've read and learned. Take a few deep breaths and relax. And read on.

To do today

Ask a family member to do something just for you, then sit back and enjoy the moment.

Meet One of the Nice Girls

Shawna now

Shawna is a forty-five-year-old black woman who looks older than her years due to health problems—diabetes and metabolic syndrome—and heavy family responsibilities. She came to therapy because she just "didn't feel like myself," and it was soon evident that she suffered from ongoing depression. At 187 pounds, she looks as if she's carrying the weight of the world with her everywhere she goes.

She has two teenage sons and a husband who was recently laid off his job due to a back injury, and she manages a home health aide agency. She hates to say no to anyone, and her boys are used to haranguing her until she gives in. They're basically decent kids but have way too much power in the family and Shawna admits that she spoils them rotten. Her husband is helpful to a point, especially since he's been the disciplinarian in the family, but currently he's depressed due to his physical limitations, not working, and having to depend on Shawna so much.

Moreover, her elderly parents who live an hour away are demanding more of her time. As they age, they're fighting more, threatening to leave each other and go live with one of their children. It upsets Shawna to see them at each other's throats and she fears refusing their requests will exacerbate their stress. Her two siblings live out of state and rely on Shawna to shoulder all the elder care responsibilities.

Most of the time in therapy Shawna doesn't know where to begin to share what's going on: If her parents don't need something done on the weekends, her kids are begging her to take them to the mall or to the movies, or her husband is in so much pain that she has to help him get in and out of a chair, or she gets "emergency" calls from work at all hours of the day. The only way she knows how to relieve her stress and anxiety is through food, but the fatter she gets, the more she hates herself. She knows she's destroying her health but says that some days, "I push it out of my mind. I just don't care."

Shawna as a child

She is the youngest child, with a brother and sister a decade older than her. Because they were both out of the house when she was still in grade school, she and her parents were very close and she grew up feeling like an only child. Her parents worked hard to get ahead, were equally strict and loving with her, and she believes she owes them a great deal for what they gave her. They spent much of her childhood bickering and blaming each other for household problems and Shawna either tried to distract them from fighting or jumped in to mediate. She believed that if she was a good girl, they'd have less to worry about and the fighting would let up. And she often sought solace through food.

Shawna did well in school but had few friends. She enjoyed coming home and doing her homework and was afraid to be away too long because she knew, even at a young age, that her parents picked at each other less when she was around. Although they weren't physically abusive with each other, Shawna admits that she never knew if their verbal assaults would someday cross the line and turn uglier. When her adult brother and sister came for visits, they seemed like fish out of water and rarely stayed longer than a few days. She couldn't understand how they could just turn off their feelings about her parents and go merrily off and live their own lives.

It took a good deal of coaxing when Shawna's husband proposed to her to get her out of the house. At first she wanted to live near her parents, but her husband insisted they move far enough away that they could have their own life. When she was younger, it was no trouble to drive back and forth to see her folks, and she often stayed overnight, leaving her kids home with her husband. With him now so helpless and with her current job pressures, that's no longer an option. Talk about being stuck between a rock and a hard place.

De-nicing Shawna

After starting antidepressants, Shawna became a little more hopeful, encouraged enough to start meeting with a registered dietician to help her make healthier food selections. In the meantime, I worked with her on finding ways to de-stress and relax, including spending numerous sessions with her and her husband focusing on improving their relationship and parenting their kids more effectively. The kids were furious at first that Mom was unwrapping herself from around their fingers, but gradually they became less entitled and demanding.

When Shawna's siblings were in town, we had a meeting. A family strategy was developed that took the weight off her as the exclusive parental caretaker. It was decided that if her siblings couldn't be there in person, they had to fork over some dough to pay for outside care. As well, both of her parents were evaluated by a geriatric care manager to assess what kinds of concrete and clinical services they needed.

Plans and strategies were only one aspect of my work with Shawna. The rest was helping her not to feel overly responsible for pleasing her children, husband, and parents. It was painful for her to back out of her parents' relationship even a bit, and she worried more about them the less she saw them. The biggest change was her feeling less stress from her children as her husband took over more of the caretaking and resumed his former disciplinary role. Shawna also learned when he really needed help and when he didn't but wanted only emotional support or simply more of her attention.

What's Next? *In Chapter 5, "Taking Care of Friends," you'l learn*

- How you choose friends who reinforce your nice girl role

- How you re-create your caretaking role in the family with friends

- What healthy friendships are made of

FIVE

Go Cry on Your Own Shoulders!

Taking Care of Friends

Friends, like family, can make you feel as if you're the luckiest gal in the world—or they can be one more category of animate objects to care for. Actually, unlike family, where fortune plays a major role in whom we end up with, having solid, supportive, there-for-you-anytime friends is hardly a matter of luck because we get to choose our friends. I've known women who've moved around the country and lived all over the world, from childhood through adulthood, and have best buddies from every place they've settled. I've also known women who find it hard to make friends, who insist there's no one around, and that people aren't open or interested in befriending them. Funny how this latter group of women nearly always winds up isolating themselves or choosing friends most of us wouldn't touch with a ten-foot licorice stick.

I'm not saying that circumstances don't play a part in hooking up with buddies. Relocating a lot, having little time to devote to socializing, or even being terribly shy can all make seeking and finding sympatico people difficult. Plus, some highly sociable women have more good friends than they know what to do with because they're so outgoing and friendly that friendships sprout up wherever they go. They're people magnets and can't help but draw folks to them.

Also, the number of buddies you have has nothing to do with the quality of friendships. Some women have a slew of acquaintances to go out and do things with—catch a play, attend a concert, see a movie, grab a quick dinner, take off on vacation—but no one to talk to about personal, intimate issues. Others have sob sisters who complain to each other about the trials and tribulations of life over coffee, drinks, or dinner, but never have the oomph to get out and do anything fun and exciting. It's important to have both kinds of buddies: those to whom you can open your heart and those whose company you value because you enjoy the same activities.

▌ **GRAB YOUR THINKING CAP** What kinds of friends do you have—acquaintances, people to do only activities with, bosom buddies who feel like sisters or brothers, sob sisters? Are you satisfied with your social network? If not, what's lacking? ▌

Don't people just fall into friendships?

It may seem as if friendships simply erupt out of the blue, but the fact is that every communication toward a person either brings you closer to or farther away from him or her. If each time you greet your new neighbor she says hello back, you've got a good chance of developing camaraderie—you tell her about your new job, she tells you about her ex-husband (or vice versa). But if you try to get chummy and she's all business, you might rightly feel the door to friendship is more closed than open. Maybe you give her a few more chances, but pretty soon you get the message that she's not in the market for a new gal pal.

▌ GRAB YOUR THINKING CAP Do you become close with people merely because they're around (at work or school, on your block, in your building, at your kid's school)? Are most of your relationships due to you intentionally seeking out another person as a friend, his or her courting you, or happenstance? ▌

The best friendships are a combination of serendipity and hard work. At a party, you're introduced to another attorney who, like you, was the only girl in a family of brothers. Or in the lunchroom, you discover that your coworker in the next cubicle lived in the same college dorm you did at the same time, but you don't have the foggiest recollection of each other. At a conference, you meet a colleague you feel drawn to because you share political values and have a sharp, quirky sense of humor. There is something that draws us to people. You might find you have a great deal in common—you both sail or ski or are history buffs. Or you admire particular aspects of a person—her ease around people, the way she put herself through college while raising three kids single-handedly, his passion for the underdog and community volunteer efforts, the way he says what he means and doesn't back down, her fantastic sense of the absurd.

If that kind of connection doesn't generally happen for you, that is, feeling drawn to someone for good and clear reasons, then it's time to start inspecting potential friends from a more rational, intentional perspective. The making of friendships should happen through a gut sense of rightness as well as using good judgment that says, here is a person who has many fine qualities, with whom I appear to have common interests and values, and who also seems to want to get to know me better.

Many women don't know how to go out and pick friends and end up sliding into relationships with whoever's available—your next-door neighbor who's always begging you to go out for a drink but ignores you once you get to a club; your colleague who can't wait to tell you the latest gossip about everyone else in the office; your fellow student who lets you copy his homework and thinks it's okay to drop by your apartment unannounced at all hours; your manicurist who wants to know everything about you but is tight-lipped about herself; the woman in your book group who makes cutting remarks about absent members but is all syrupy sweetness to their face; the guy at the gym who laments his sorry life but asks no questions about you.

Are you picking up the thread here? Can you see the red flags in each example: your Jekyll-and-Hyde neighbor, gossipy colleague, intrusive and unethical fellow student, nosy manicurist, two-faced book group comrade, and narcissistic victim of a gym buddy? Each one might as well be marching around with a neon sign that says, "Probably not good friendship material." No matter how many other terrific qualities a person has, from the get-go you need to watch out for what you can already see that might spoil the relationship. Should you avoid a snap judgment and spend a little time with someone to determine what she's like? Absolutely. Then, either the relationship will become more or less enjoyable and satisfying. My opinion: Get to know everyone a little, then pursue people who are worthwhile and sympatico—and who aren't draped in red flags. Better to be alone than with someone who's not worthy of your friendship.

■ **GRAB YOUR THINKING CAP** Do you miss red flags that indicate people may not be suitable friendship material? Why don't you see them? Is it willful blindness, do ya think? ▪

If my current friends aren't the cream of the crop, should I dump 'em and start fresh?

There are two approaches you can take to assessing friendships and what to do with them. The first is to ask yourself, Does my circle of friends meet my social and emotional needs? Start by wondering, On the whole, do I have enough intimates whom I'd die for and who'd die for me (okay, that's a bit over the top, but you get the gist)? I'm talking about sacred sisters (or brothers) who have proved themselves over and over and are just about the most spectacular friends anyone on the planet could ever wish for. You want to have at least one, if not two or three of these. I know that's a tall order, but it helps to have more, rather than fewer, close friends. In spite of cell phone accessibility, friends occasionally deserve private time and do drift out of signal range.

The next step is to consider if you have enough people in your life who share your passions, values, and interests. Can you count on people to enjoy doing what you like to do, and vice versa, so that you can stay socially engaged and have fun? This is not an idle question. Too many nice girls work hard and don't know how to play. They turn food into fun instead of pursuing more satisfying activities. If your best friend is in Aruba on vacation, she may be available on the phone to cheer you up when you get the flu, but she's not about to wing it home to take in a special watercolor exhibit. You need at least a handful of people who have similar interests or who are easygoing and happy to join you in your plans. They may not be a disco diva like you, but they'll tag along to a dance club. Or even though they're not wild about opera, they'll join you because they can't pass up a chance to dress up.

Okay, that's the general approach to evaluating friendships. Now listen up for strategy number two: Consider each of your friends individually—your former roommates, sorority sisters, old college chums, people you hang with from work, coffee-klatch neighbors, kids' friends' parents, gym buddies, and your oldest friend from second grade. Go through them one by one and decide if you value the friendship, including why or why not. I know, right about now you're dreaming about how scrumptious a chocolate chip cookie would taste, but bear with me. I didn't say analyzing friendships would be a piece of cake. So tick off all the people on your list and decide if they're worthy of you and whether you love having them in your life.

My guess is that you'll find some friends who receive a resounding yes, some who make your heart sink, and others who make you shrug or feel pulled in two directions. All natural and normal. However, if everyone on your list makes you gag or yawn, or even if most of your crew only elicits a shrug, you're in big trouble. Sadly, some of us have only old friends whom we would not in a million years pick now. In fact, how many of your friends would you choose again? I'm serious; count 'em up. The fact that you have little in common with them now but enjoy a shared history is not necessarily a reason to dump them. As long as you're still more satisfied than not with the relationship, it's a keeper. If you have a bunch of great buddies and a few people who don't make the "choose again" list, that's okay.

Pay special attention to the alleged friends who don't make the grade *because they fail to hold up their end of the friendship*. Maybe they have lots of other close friends or other time or social commitments, are self-centered, or are in your life through a mutual friend who has since moved on. Maybe they're chronically depressed but refuse to do anything about it. (An aside about people who suffer from depression. This certainly is not a reason to avoid or disavow a friendship. People go through rough patches and can't be there for you at times because they have their own troubles. But there are friends who have depression and still maintain a friendship and others who simply do not have the energy or interest to connect or give back. Only you know how much of a drain they are and whether they're doing everything possible to help themselves get and stay better. If they're not, well, you can probably guess what I have to say about having too many of them on your dance card.)

If someone doesn't ring your chimes, why are you wasting your time with him or her? Having a bunch of friends who don't take care of you emotionally is not a neutral situation. I'm not talking about having high expectations of people you see only at the annual holiday party or folks you go out for a drink with once every quarter after a board meeting. You wouldn't expect acquaintances like these to be your safety net. But people who purport to be good friends and are not do emotional damage when each time you reach out to them they're not there for you.

▌ **GRAB YOUR THINKING CAP** What did you learn from assessing your friendships—are you all set, do you need to reflect more on the subject, are you shocked that you thought you were in great shape with friends and aren't? ▌

What about friendships that start out like wildfire, then sputter out?

Sometimes you meet someone and you get on like a house on fire. You're on the phone with each other every free minute, can't wait 'til the next time you get together, and feel as if your life has changed just by knowing each other. The feeling is infatuation, similar to what you experience with a lover or someone you're romantically interested in. You think your instant buddy is special, one in a million, and she feels the same way; such a sensation is heady and exciting. Often, these wildfires burn down to a steady low flame and you continue to warm each other's hearts for years to come. The mutuality, pleasure, sharing, and interdependence deepen and you've made a friend for life. When I say, "Lucky you!" I mean it; close friends are an absolute treasure.

However, sometimes the initial blaze masks relational dysfunction, an unconscious need for each other that isn't healthy. You're swept up in your friend's tragic life story and see yourself as her savior; she requires a great deal of attention and you become her salvation. Actually, the motivations of relationship are not generally this clear (unless you're someone who reflects a great deal on her behavior). Things just feel right (that is, familiar): Your urge to take care of what's frail and fragile intersects with your friend's need to be taken care of. The fit feels perfect, but it's all wrong.

Things go awry when you find yourself doing more and more (and her doing less and less) and going overboard in the care department. You may be confused by why you're not feeling the same way you used to and find yourself starting to resent her. So you redouble your efforts. She may sense your desire to pull back and, therefore, start easing off the relationship in fear of you dropping her. Even if the relationship gets back on an even keel, sooner or later her neediness and your overdoing will crowd out whatever else is healthy and positive in the relationship.

Because friendship isn't a science, it's difficult to measure the balance of give-and-take. You want to avoid a tit-for-tat situation—*you need to pay for the phone call this week because I paid last week*—but you also don't want to be doing all the heavy lifting while your friend is busy filing her nails. You want to cultivate and establish a felt sense of equilibrium and fairness. Sometimes you may need help figuring out what's going on and require feedback from family and other friends. If you trust the people you generally go to for advice, listen carefully to what they have to say. Many times everyone else in your circle can see that you're being used but you. If that's the general consensus, take off your blinders or watch out: You're about to be taken down by your own good heart.

Sometimes friendships fizzle out because neither party has the communication skills to address and fix problems—and there are difficulties for even the best of friends. In fact, weathering difficulties is exactly what cements relationships. If a friend hurts you and you don't speak up but expect her to read your mind, you're setting up the relationship to fail. If two friends are both shy about expressing their needs, how can a relationship get over the bumps? Friendships also fizzle because of the limits of individuals. There's a phase that two-year-olds go through called parallel play in which they engage in activities side by side but there's no real connection between them. Adults often have similar kinds of playmates: people to go places with but with whom there is no real attachment or intimacy. Over dinner, you talk about your week and she talks about hers without any meeting of the minds or hearts. This kind of relationship has a short shelf life because, as the saying goes, there's no there there!

▮ **GRAB YOUR THINKING CAP** Who is generally the caretaker in your friendships, you or your friends? Do you have virtual, parallel play relationships with no depth? Is it hard to get past rough patches because you're unable to share hurt feelings and you pick friends with a similar disability? ▮

So what makes for a healthy friendship?

A healthy friendship is like any other relationship, encouraging you to flourish and making you feel better and better about knowing the other person. Yes, yes, yes, there are times when you will wonder what you're doing being friends with someone: She's sooooo picky about restaurants, his indecisiveness drives you up a wall, she's obsessed with Baroque music and you're a hard-rock gal, why can't he just settle down in one place rather than moving around the country every few years, she never reads the newspaper and couldn't care less about politics. The reason you have differences is that you are separate people.

The goal is not to eradicate differences but to resolve or live with them. How you do this is key. Friends should care that they upset you (of course, you have to tell them first, now, don't you?) and try their hardest not to offend. They should show as much interest in you as you do in them, be willing to compromise, and there should be an easy, comfortable give-and-take between you. One of the most vital things friends do is create safety for mutual sharing. You need to trust each other emotionally and allow yourself to be authentic, which means validating each other and giving honest, tactful feedback. Most important, especially for nice girls, is—drumroll, please—you should be taking excellent emotional care of each other. In a solid friendship, there's a sense of parity, reciprocity, roughly equal contribution, not because you each give the same amount but because, over time, your efforts balance out.

If you don't have this kind of friendship with at least a few people in your life, no wonder you're a ball of stress. Not only is there no one to talk with honestly about your problems, but you're probably taking on *other* people's messes, creating a double load for yourself. That's why being able both to care for others *and* be taken care of is essential. Dependence reduces stress, which, lest we forget this book is about eating, lessens your inclination to turn to food when you're in emotional turmoil.

One of the saddest parts of my job is meeting clients who never have had a positive, healthy relationship. True intimacy is too scary or unfamiliar, or requires skills they don't have. Many awfully nice women will pay a professional to act like a friend and unburden themselves to the hilt, but wouldn't think of sharing the details of their lives with a peer. That tells me they are fairly certain that a therapist will take them seriously and hear them out but don't trust someone they're not paying to do the same job. How heartbreaking is that?

Okay, in case you're not sure where your buddies stand on the friendometer, here are some questions that should give you answers. A word of caution: It may be hard to acknowledge that you've been a doormat or a patsy, that you're easily taken in and as easily cast off, that you've given more than you've received. This is no time for remorse and regrets. You can flagellate yourself later (but I hope you won't). For now, just be honest, nonjudgmental, and curious about your responses. You didn't set out to be taken advantage of; you simply haven't had the proper skills and attitude needed to sift out the gold from the garbage. You're learning. So be it.

As you read through these questions, think on two tracks: your sense of your friendships in general and your relationships with each individual you call friend.

- Do you spend a good deal of time listening to friends' problems?

- Do you repeatedly give advice that isn't taken and hear the same complaints week after week (or, worse, year after year)?

- Are you assiduous about keeping commitments (dinners, concerts, movies, etc.) but find friends don't share the same diligence and often break dates for frivolous reasons?

- Do you generally remember to send cards or give gifts for friends' special occasions, while they forget or have pathetic excuses for not acknowledging yours?

- Do you have friends who feel free to "be honest" and say whatever they want even if it hurts you, but get all huffy when you give them the slightest bit of negative feedback?

- Are your friends two-faced and do they talk about you behind your back?

- Do your friends betray confidences and tell your secrets for no good reason?

- Do your friends go that extra mile for you the same way you do for them?

- Do you have conversations with friends in which they never ask how you are or what you're up to?

- Must you think the way a friend does or she has a hissy fit, gives you the cold shoulder, or puts you down?

- Do your friends support what's in *your* best interest even if it conflicts with *theirs*?

- Are friends on-again, off-again, that is, best buddy one moment, impossible to track down even with a bloodhound and a private eye the next?

If you're dissatisfied with the quality or quantity of current friendships, don't despair. As you quit throwing yourself into being nice and start evaluating people on whether they deserve your ever-lovin' largesse, there'll be a sea change in your relationships. You may end up losing some alleged friends, but that will make room for authentic intimates. Remember, if you're making do, you may not be open to meeting new people who have more to offer you.

Making friends is work. It means being on the lookout for your kind of person, then thinking in terms of a probationary period when potential chums need to prove themselves worthy of you. I don't mean you have to scrutinize and analyze their every move. However, I am saying that you have to keep your eyes wide open to red flags and keep testing them. Watch how they treat people, learn about their other friendships (past and current), pay exquisite attention to how you feel when you're with them (and when you're not). If you feel anxious around them, something is wrong, as is also true if you feel an ongoing longing for approval and a desire to please them at all costs. That is not the stuff of real, lasting friendship. Friendships bring out the best in you and make your life easier, not harder.

How does my niceness regarding friends drive me to eat?

There are a few ways you can get yourself into trouble here. First, by not having enough companions and confidants, food becomes your best buddy. Instead of calling on Connie, Alicia, Steve, or Shana to help you sort out a mess you got yourself into or to pull you up and out of the doldrums you've been in ever since your last fling ended badly, you surround yourself with chums named Ben, Jerry, Uncle Ben, Mrs. Smith, and Sara Lee. Whenever you regularly substitute food for people because you don't have enough intimates in your life or because you fear burdening or depending on others, something is seriously wrong. Your choices keep you isolated and give you no real help. In fact, they compound your problems.

Another way dysfunctional relationships propel you in the direction of your pantry is that by not depending on people, you overstress yourself. And you know where you turn for soothing and solace when that happens. Due to your quest not to make waves or enemies and be all things to all people, the pressure becomes so unbearable that you reach out to the closest thing available when you're about to explode—food. You need instant gratification and comfort and there it is beckoning to you from so many cute little bags and boxes. By allowing yourself to become overstressed, you set yourself up for a fall—off the wagon and into the cheese dip.

One final way that seriously flawed friendships may cause you to seek out sweets and treats is how your networks view eating and weight. In certain circles, food and fat are the enemy and, trying to fit in, you may place yourself in a position of trying to lose weight too fast or become thinner than your body should be. Pressure to be included can be intense and, rather than friends helping you to become comfortable with your body, you may be surrounding yourself with people who subtly and not so subtly give you the message that you need to be fit to fit in. Conversely, if your friendships are cemented by food and revolve around eating, you may not have the guts to try to make some changes in what you do when you're hanging out or to break away from the old gang. You may be too frightened that you'll hurt feelings or that people will think you're selfish or arrogant just because you want to take care of yourself!

NO MORE NICE GIRL MANIFESTO FOR FRIENDS

DO

- Extend yourself toward people you like and care about.

- Expect friends to be emotionally healthy, self-aware, and working on resolving their issues.

- Require that friends be good listeners, go out of their way for you, provide validation, understanding, sound advice, and solicited (and if you are harming yourself, unsolicited) feedback.

- Seek out people who can put aside their needs and desires and who have your interest at heart.

- Encourage friends to share their honest feelings with you in a tactful, appropriate way, even if their words hurt.

- Anticipate that communicating authentically with friends does not come automatically but takes time, commitment, trust, guts, and energy.

- Surround yourself with people who can take feedback so that you don't have to sit on your hurt and stuff your feelings with food.

- Have enough friends that all your eggs aren't in one basket and have different kinds of associations for varying needs and activities (going out, heart-to-heart talks, etc.).

- Allow that friends aren't perfect and neither are you.

- Expect that friends will share equally the work of forging a spectacular relationship.

- Know that you will make and lose friends throughout life and believe that you will always have good friends as long as you want and seek them out.

DON'T

- Keep friends just because you feel bad for them or are afraid to cut them loose.

- Accept ongoing excuses from people who cannot live up to your reasonable expectations about friendship.

- Keep on doing for people who don't give back to you in return.

- Take an ongoing part in relationships in which a friend wants you to be her mother, can't admit to being wrong, is a perpetual victim, or has to have the last word.

- Wear blinders, ignore red flags, or avoid seeing the truth about alleged friends.

- Believe you don't need friends and can take care of yourself emotionally without them.

- Spend a lot of time with people you don't enjoy or who don't add to your life.

- Try to fix friends' problems; instead support them in fixing their own problems.

- Let other people pressure you into staying friends with someone for his own reasons when it is not in your best interest.

- Pal around with people who aren't introspective and self-reflective, can't laugh at themselves, and refuse to go into therapy if they have severe dysfunctions.

- Keep company with friends who see themselves as living under a black cloud, because they'll only make you feel helpless and push you into a caretaking role.

Well, that's it. Another area of your life has gone under the microscope and you've survived. You now know how to sidestep being too nice with family and friends. Of course, you can't go out and make all the changes you need to de-nice yourself and improve your relationship with food today, but you've got tomorrow and the day after and the day after that.

To do today

Call a person who you'd like to get to know or get to know better to say hello.

Meet One of the Nice Girls

Clarice now

Clarice is a sixty-six-year-old single, retired teacher, referred to me by her cardiologist after she was diagnosed with minor heart problems that she assumes are due to stress. Stress? What could possibly be stressful about desperately wanting to be loved by everyone? Clarice has a self-admitted "heart of gold that gets me into trouble." In her groups of friends, she's the hostess for every party, the chauffeur for whoever needs to be driven to the hospital or picked up at the airport, the shoulder for every victim to cry on, and the bank for every girlfriend who needs a loan. Good thing she's retired—she'd never have time for a job.

When I ask Clarice if friends do as much for her as she does for them, she either shrugs or changes the subject. It's enormously hard for her to stop giving and start taking. She explains that it's genetic, that her mother and two sisters are exactly the same way. The few times she's talked honestly about her fears, she admits to "not wanting to disappoint people." When I ask which people, she shrugs again—anyone and everyone. She's rarely bothered about letting herself down and wouldn't have come to see me if she didn't have problems with her ticker.

Her favorite trait about herself is that she's a good listener, and she really is—she listens to all her friends' problems and gives advice that could probably put me out of business if she chose to turn professional. Clarice is one sharp cookie, with amazing insights into friends' dilemmas and difficulties. However, she has little interest in applying her shrink skills to understanding herself and improving her life. Every time she shows me a bit of Clarice, she looks embarrassed, then does some fancy footwork to dance off to a different subject.

Clarice can't remember a time when she was a "normal" weight. She recalls being a plump child and adolescent who "ballooned up" in college and has never been less than size fourteen. Although she insists she wants to lose weight, she loves to cook as much as she loves to eat. Playing chef is one of the few ways she takes care of herself. Although she's not a junk food eater, she adores pastries, pasta, aged cheeses, and creamy sauces. It's difficult to get Clarice to talk about the feelings that distress her, but I know that underneath her pleasant exterior she is lonely, perhaps depressed, and emotionally uncomfortable when she's not busy taking care of others.

Clarice as a child

Like many nice girls, Clarice grew up with an alcoholic parent: her mother. Clarice's two younger sisters have already died, one from diabetes and the other from alcoholism. Her father worked first as a painter, then as a school janitor. Her mother had been a teacher who did her job during the day, but "drank pretty steadily" every night. Clarice, her mother, and sisters all enjoyed cooking and had great times together in the kitchen preparing lavish dinners. After dinner, it was Clarice's job to care for her sisters and put them to bed, then do the same for her mother while her father either watched TV or read the newspaper.

Family members didn't talk much, if at all, about feelings. Had Clarice and her sisters discussed Mom's drinking and Dad's indifference, she might have understood that she wasn't alone in her distress. But Clarice believed it was her duty to protect her sisters from pain and unhappiness, and she bore the family burden herself. If she enjoyed anything at home aside from cooking, it was the feeling of being in charge and valued. She knew (or believed she knew) that without her, the family would fall apart.

De-nicing Clarice

Clarice and I talked a lot about the trade-offs of taking care of her friends versus herself. The hardest work with her was her almost total disconnection from and discomfort with distressing feelings. Slowly she began to identify emotions: She *did* feel a bit taken advantage of, she *did* wish deep down that her friends would reciprocate once in a while, she *did* yearn for someone to lean on. Of course, every time we touched on one of these subjects, it hit a nerve that snaked back into her past— her mother and, to a lesser extent, her father. They weren't there for her emotionally, so she fell into three patterns: burying her feelings by giving others what *she* needed (love, care, attention, etc.), pretending that she was so strong and capable that she didn't have needs to begin with, and turning to food in order not to feel.

One of the best things Clarice did was commit to going to the gym. She found a place near her and went religiously. Although she didn't note any major weight changes initially, she started to see that it was okay to do something for herself and still be there for others. In fact, once she got into it, she brought two friends along with her. We tackled her eating problems by focusing on why and when she ate through a feelings log, which she also kept consistently. Slowly she began to see that much of her cooking and eating frenzies were attempts to ward off uncomfortable feelings of disappointment, loneliness, dissatisfaction with life in general. Not surprising, when she began to feel more, she began to eat less.

What's Next? *In Chapter 6, "Taking Care at Work,"*
you'll learn

- How you set yourself up for overdoing with colleagues
  and your boss

- How to overcome your tendency to caretake on the job

- How to avoid unhealthy eating at work

SIX

Do I Look Like
Santa's Helper?

Taking Care at Work

Hi, ho, hi, ho, it's off to work you go. The place where you probably spend about half your waking hours. Unless you can do your job utterly alone and hardly ever come into contact with another soul, as a niceaholic you have to watch out for overdoing. If you're not dealing with bosses, colleagues, and subordinates, you have suppliers, distributors, and clients likely to channel the Mother Teresa in you.

There are a host of ways you can overdo niceness at work, almost all of which involve a constitutional inability to pronounce audibly the simplest of monosyllabic words: "no." Sometimes you'd swear you were thinking no, and are stunned when yes inexplicably pops out of your mouth. Other times, you find yourself vigorously nodding before someone has even finished making a request or demand. Fortunately, this book will give you the tools you need to outgrow those self-destructive urges.

So why can't you help saying yes at work or shake behavior that consistently gets you into trouble by ramping up your stress level? The answer is simple: Work is not only a microcosm of how you interact in the larger world but also a loose replica of that old template established by growing up in your family of origin within a hierarchical social structure. Remember, a template lays down patterns that quickly turn into habitual behavior and automatic responses. Working in any group setting—small office, large corporation, hospital, school, civil service, etc.—it's natural to react unconsciously as you did in your formative years. The family is your very first social group; every formal and informal association of people ever after has the ability to evoke the original template—for good or bad.

Here's an example. Say your father was a rageful son of a gun who brooked no challenges, and the way you learned to survive in family boot camp was to remain invisible and zip your lip. You either stayed in your room or out of the house, spent a great deal of time in your head, and tried to keep under Dad's radar as much as possible. Fast-forward a few decades and here you are working for a Cruella De Vil who always has to have the last word and rips apart anyone who dares confront her. What feelings might she evoke in you? How do you think you'll react when the two of you have a difference of opinion and your boss pitches a fit? My money's on you freezing, slithering away with a stunned look on your face, or maybe retreating to your office to lose yourself in gleeful fantasies of revenge while rooting through your desk drawers to find that package of M&M's you stashed away last August.

The fact is that unless someone has had substantial therapy and worked her butt off doing a personality makeover, she's going to respond on the job the same way she acted in her family. And if that behavior involved making nice, because not making nice was going to land her in the doghouse, that's what she'll do.

▌ GRAB YOUR THINKING CAP Are you a yes-girl at work? Can you see how your upbringing shaped you into one? How do you feel about yourself when you don't swallow your real feelings? How do you feel about yourself when you do? ▌

If I start speaking up at work and get fired, will you support me?

Uh, 'fraid not, but the question does speak to your ultimate fear about being assertive. Because experience tells us unequivocally that nice tends to elicit approval and not nice tends to provoke censure, most of us know just how to get our bread buttered. An emotionally healthy person enjoys approval and tries to be nice, but also knows that she can withstand disapproval for good cause. She does whatever is in her best interest most of the time, which means recognizing that she's going to upset or piss off some people when she says no.

However, that's not the kind of socialization that produces nice girls like you. You're nice because you're afraid to be naughty. If you were unfortunate enough to have a parent (or two) who treated you unfairly—punished, rejected, or abandoned you physically or emotionally—because he or she didn't approve of what you had to say, you were conditioned to be nice. If refusing demands or requests brought on negative consequences, if challenging authority resulted in withdrawal of love and affection, if thinking for yourself led to alienation of affection, humiliation, or exclusion from the family unit, you adapted and went along to get along. You were in survival mode, a darned good choice at the time.

The problem is that even though you now may have a string of credentials after your name and may be a rising star in or at the top of your field, you still feel like a three-year-old inside and are terrified to rock the boat at work and most other places. Even though your boss, colleagues, or subordinates may be half your age, around them you're still reacting from that kid inside you who so badly wants love and approval that you'll sacrifice good sense and good self-care to get it. A bigger problem is that most of the time you're not even aware that the child in you is running the show. How can you rewrite the script if you're oblivious of the plot and how the characters interact?

I'm not saying that speaking up is always the best option. The idea is to have a range of choices and pick the one that will be most effective in a situation. There's a big difference between telling your sweetheart of a boss that you can't do a top-notch job alone and need some help and raising the issue with a supervisor who's not your biggest fan and who's in the midst of choosing which supervisee to lay off due to budget cuts. The key here is options: You have the ability to speak up but use your judgment to decide when and where. Nice girls aren't comfortable asserting themselves and are almost always living in protection or survival mode, even when they no longer need to.

Exactly how do I overdo the nice thing at work when I shouldn't?

Let me count the ways. Unfortunately, there are quite a number of them. Again, let me remind you that doing your fair share and even going overboard once in a while are desirable traits in

an employee. Putting in an extra hour here or there, volunteering, or occasionally taking on an odious task that no one wants
to do shows initiative, spunk, passion, team spirit, drive, lead-
ership, and commitment to your job. If you do these things for
the right reasons, you feel proud of yourself and other people
will rightfully admire you and might even view you as a role
model. What you want to avoid, however, is earning the label
of chump, self-sacrificer, angel, soft touch, or Saint Arlene.

Here are some work traps in which nice girls become all too
easily ensnared. They're interrelated and have a great deal in
common because they're based on false assumptions and un-
founded fears. If you recognize yourself, please don't reach for
the leather strap. Better that you chuckle or feel sad about how
you've been hurting yourself all these years than get down
on behavior that started out as adaptive and that you've been
using to survive because you haven't known how to manage
more effectively.

You can't say no to requests or demands without feeling guilty

This is one of your major problems and causes you untold
amounts of stress. Most of the decisions in your life—in and
out of work—are driven by guilt, or fear of feeling guilty,
which is a kamikaze way to operate. Instead, you need to respond logically to requests or demands by asking yourself: Do
I have the time, energy, ability, resources, or interest in meeting this request or demand? What are the real consequences if
I say yes? What are the real (not imagined) consequences if I
say no? You can't possibly analyze a situation rationally when
every fiber of your being is terrified of letting someone down
and failing to live up to your ridiculously perfectionist standards, and when your main drive is to steer clear of conflict
and emotional distress.

Think about the way you set yourself up: If you can't stand to feel guilty, you'll never say no unless your back is against the wall—as in you're totally incapacitated and unable to move or speak. Of course, knowing you, you'll blink out "y-e-s" right before your last, dying breath. Seriously, to act in your best interest when someone wants something from you, you have two effective choices: either you learn to say no *without* feeling guilty or you learn to say it and tolerate the guilt. Both options are acceptable and each works like a charm.

The way you learn not to feel guilty is to analyze a situation rationally and decide if guilt is a suitable reaction, so listen up. *The emotion of guilt is appropriate only when you have done something wrong.* If your boss asks you to stay late and you've got opera tickets and refuse, you're doing nothing wrong or bad (unless the fate of the world is at stake). He may *think* you're a lousy employee or a selfish person, but would the average person? Would I? Of course not. You have to stop and answer this question: Am I doing something that most healthy people would think is wrong or bad? If so, then guilt is appropriate; if not, chuck it.

The second way to feel okay about refusing requests and demands is to tolerate feeling guilty—for a while. Maybe your boss asks you to stay late, but you really want to get home because you've worked late two nights straight. You say no and feel bad all the way home. Okay, how long are you going to court guilt? All night? For the rest of the week? For the rest of your life? Of course not. So you feel a little guilty, so what? Like gas, it'll pass. We can't be all things to all people and a smidgen of guilt won't kill you or anyone else.

You need to figure out why guilt is such a hot button for you and why you're so afraid of it. Ladies, we're not talking about being dragged out and shot at dawn. *That's* something to be afraid of; an emotion isn't. It'll visit and it'll go away. If it doesn't move along on its own, give it a nudge and keep pushing 'til it's gone. Guilt is hardly a fatal disease or a condition you're stuck with for life. It's an intense emotion that comes and goes and that you can choose to welcome or kick out the door.

▌ **GRAB YOUR THINKING CAP** How hard is it to say no to requests and demands at work because you feel guilty or fear you will? Why else don't you say no more often? ▌

You think you have to do everything yourself

If you don't have a cape stitched to your clavicles, you're not Superwoman, so why insist on doing everything at work yourself? What's wrong with sharing the load, delegating, giving someone else a chance to learn what you know? What's wrong is that doing so causes you to feel so anxious that you tell yourself you can't bear it. Somewhere along the way (in your family growing up, actually), you learned that you can't depend on other people and must do everything yourself if you want the job done or done right.

You'd secretly love to get help but are petrified to give up control because you believe all hell will break loose. Okay, maybe your parents weren't always on top of things, but that was then and this is now. Think about it: Are your employees, supervisees, or colleagues really such nitwits that you can't trust them to do their jobs? Aren't there at least a couple of them who can walk and chew gum at the same time? You need to assess your situation rationally, particularly who has what skills and whether there's a reality-based, concrete reason to do everything yourself. More likely, your fears are getting in the way of striking a balance between holding on to control and letting it go.

The worst thing that can happen when you delegate or cede

control is that someone doesn't do a great job or the same job that you would. In your head, you might imagine catastrophe, but it's unlikely that you're surrounded by total nincompoops. If you are, then you don't belong where you're working. No one should remain in a job in which she is truly the only one capable of making wise decisions and getting things done. It's a setup for your stressometer (and your blood pressure) to soar off the charts. It's also a setup for you to feed your face.

█ GRAB YOUR THINKING CAP Do you need to control situations at work, fear delegating or sharing work, and believe no one can do as good a job as you do? █

Even though it stresses the heck out of you, you love being the go-to person

Sure, the downside of being action central at work is exhaustion, feeling overwhelmed, and boosting your spirits with Twinkies. But, oh, the upside—everyone telling you what a marvelous, totally amazing person you are because of all you do. The adoration and the rush from all that praise could become downright addictive. I'm serious. Once we get used to being one-dimensionally valued for being overly nice, it's hard to give up all the adoration that accompanies martyrdom. In fact, the need for that good feeling may underlie much of your altruism and self-sacrifice. Rather than your big heart, it may be your desperate yearning for admiration that makes you such a shining star.

Again, if you were a parentified child growing up, you might have kept at it because of the attention you received for getting straight A's in school, taking care of a litter of siblings, and keeping the house in tiptop shape because your parents needed your help. You might have wanted to slack off and even may have tried to but found you missed the praise and compliments. There's nothing wrong with what you did then—you did what you had to do to obtain parental approval and love—but there's something wrong if you can't give up the need for admiration now when overdoing is pushing you over the edge.

■ **GRAB YOUR THINKING CAP** Fess up. Do you secretly love being seen as a goddess of goodness at work? Are you addicted to praise for overdoing? ▮

You have to be twice as good as men

At times we may wish that we lived in a nonsexist (and nonracist, nonhomophobic, etc.) society, but the fact is we don't. Women are still the main family caretakers, even if they do paid work as well. That means we usually have more on our plates than men do. Sure, he'll pick up the kids after school or put them to bed, but women are generally the ones who take off work when the little ones are sick and who do the bulk of household chores as a matter of course. Unfortunately or fortunately, we're hardwired to be pretty terrific at multitasking.

Not only is our physical and mental energy divided more than that of men, but we're still trying to prove ourselves in the workplace. Would that it weren't so, but it is. When the number of doctors, lawyers, corporate presidents, legislators, directors of boards, and heads of nations are equally balanced between men and women, we'll know we've arrived and won't have to keep busting our patoots to be perceived as merely keeping up. Until then, we'll probably feel an inner pressure to measure up or excel. If you've chosen a profession in which sexism abounds (overtly or covertly), the need to be viewed as a peer with men is a reality and will likely add stress to your life.

However, be careful that trying to be as good as or better than the guys doesn't translate into going overboard and killing yourself unnecessarily. If demands on you are so great that all you want to do is come home and dive into a Boston cream pie, you need to ask yourself if this is the right job—or career—for you. Some professions are intensely demanding no matter what gender you are, and are not for everyone. If you have trouble setting limits and feel compelled to overachieve, you'll probably be drawn to these occupations, but that doesn't mean they're good for you or your relationship with food.

If you're constantly trying to prove that you're the best, nicest, most competent person in your workplace, watch out. Frankly, if you regularly find yourself trying to prove how good you are to anyone, something is very wrong. The only person whose approval you need is your own. Stressing yourself out to prove your worth to other people, along with wanting to be perfect, only keeps you in excess mode. If you can't set and work toward realistic goals in your job, you may need to reflect on whether your standards (or company standards) are compromising your health. If eating is a reaction to overdoing on the job, it may be a signal not only that you need other ways to de-stress but that you also need to get out of a work situation that requires too much of you to live a healthy, normal life.

▎**GRAB YOUR THINKING CAP** Are you in a profession or job in which you need or feel you need to work harder than men to be perceived as doing well? What kind of toll does that take on you? Are the standards in your workplace too high, or are they realistic? ▎

You don't take credit when credit is due

Women who are too nice have a tendency to feel grossly uncomfortable taking compliments and praise, never mind whooping it up over their achievements. While humility is an admirable quality, it needs to be balanced out with being tickled pink when you've done something exceptional (or even just pretty darned good). The problem stems from early training to be modest and observing female role models—in reality, on TV, in movies—who demur and hand off credit to other people (usually men) and are, therefore, viewed as sweet and humble. Poppycock! While there's nothing wrong with sharing credit or even occasionally having an *Aw, shucks* reaction, as a modus operandi in the workplace, it's a disaster for women.

Nice women are often afraid of being perceived as boastful, conceited, full of themselves, and overly prideful. Trust me, nice women do not *ever* have to worry about getting a swelled head. A shrunken head, yes; swelled, no way.

In a healthy upbringing, children are taught to take credit and enjoy feeling good about their achievements, but not brag and lord them over others. Parents encourage progeny to enjoy success and tolerate and learn from failure. In some unhealthy environments, parents are competitive with their children. Maybe Mom was insecure and couldn't stand someone showering you with compliments because it made her feel diminished. To avoid competing, you learned to pipe down and shrug off your successes; worse, you learned to feel ashamed of being proud. Maybe you had siblings who weren't as clever as you, so you had to pretend not to do well or play down your accomplishments just so you wouldn't outshine them.

However you arrived at the place where taking credit is more pain than pleasure, you've got to turn around your thinking or you won't get over your nice girl or eating problems. Somehow in your mind it's better to come home from work and celebrate a promotion with a chunk of cheesecake than to go out and celebrate with a cadre of friends. This is not healthy behavior and, frankly, it's not even fun. Learning how to feel proud of your achievements is one of the joys of work—and living. You're bound to make plenty of mistakes along the way to balance out successes, so why not enjoy them while you can?

▌ **GRAB YOUR THINKING CAP** Are you praise/compliment/ credit aversive? How do you react to them? Do you understand what makes you so uncomfortable? ▐

What behaviors get me into trouble being too nicey-nice at work?

Now you're talking. There are specific behaviors as well as general tendencies you need to be aware of. Some of them you probably know already—quick, name two—but in case you're stumped, here are questions to help you assess where you go wrong:

- When no one volunteers for a task, are you so uncomfortable that you pipe up and say you'll do it?

- Do you pick up other people's slack on a regular basis (and not claim credit for it, to boot)?

- Do you frequently cancel plans in order to work?

- No matter how much you do at work, does it feel as if you're never doing enough?

- Do you feel overworked and undervalued because you're too nice and back off from making waves in order to do less and earn more?

- Are you scared of asking for help because you'll be perceived as weak, lazy, or incompetent?

- Do you ask for help in such a way that it sounds like you really don't want it?

- Do you beg when you should request and request when you should demand?

- As much as you hate to admit it, do you adore being the go-to person at work and having people think you're Superwoman?

- Do you think about food all day long or find you can't wait to get home from work (or go out to lunch or on break) in order to eat?

- Are you secretly furious when others claim/get credit for work you've done but keep your feelings to yourself?

- Do you feel responsible for problems at work and for making sure that everyone gets along and everything runs smoothly? (If you are top dog, that's a different story.)

How does being overly nice at work make me pack on the pounds?

I bet if you think a bit on this question, you'll come up with an answer. Picture yourself at work and stressed out of your mind with reports and deadlines, your boss looking over your shoulder, and not enough hours in the day to get everything done. Now picture yourself getting hungry or lunchtime arriving. Do you chuck all the pressure and take your salad or sandwich outside or go to the lounge to eat in peace and quiet, perhaps with your favorite CD or book? Do you spend half your lunch break enjoying eating and the rest taking a pleasant stroll or chatting with a treasured colleague? Of course not. You either gobble food while you're working or forgo it altogether.

When you're bursting with stress because you've taken

on too much and can't set limits or have to do every piece of work perfectly, you set yourself up for abusing food and your body. If you eat while you're working, you probably inhale the food and feel unsatisfied when you're done, or overeat and feel stuffed. If you postpone feeding hunger, you create a situation in which it continues to grow and grow until you're ready to eat the hair off your arm. And just what kind of food choices are you going to make when you're starving? Poor ones. And how are you going to eat those poor choices? In an unconscious feeding frenzy. Catch my drift?

Another way that work causes eating malfunctions is due to the underlying feelings of anger, resentment, helplessness, and powerlessness when you're unhappy there (even when it's your own doing!). When you're nursing one long grievance against your boss, coworkers, or the system in which you work, you're always on edge and frustrated. Feeling undervalued, taken advantage of, and put upon does not make for healthy, pleasurable eating moments. Instead of stewing and chewing, you *could* ask to see your boss about lightening your load. But, honestly, isn't it more likely that on the way to her office you'll get sidelined by the snack machine and end up snarfing down a couple of packages of Tostitos instead?

NO MORE NICE GIRL MANIFESTO AT WORK

DO

• Think long and hard before responding to requests and demands.

• Ask others for help when you need it without worrying what they'll think of you.

- Enjoy your achievements and successes and take credit for them.

- Stop feeling guilty when you say no.

- Risk not getting approval if you need to confront or challenge someone.

- Find outside people to help you establish a realistic perspective of your work attitude and behavior.

- Change jobs or careers if yours is too stressful.

- Recognize that it's not your job to solve everyone's problems at work.

- Acknowledge that you're allowed to be imperfect and make mistakes.

- Realize that you'll have to make changes slowly to see where they will lead you.

- Seek self-approval over other approval.

- Let everyone be responsible for herself or himself.

- Take all your vacation time and stay home when you're sick or exhausted.

DON'T

- Automatically say yes because you think it's expected of you.

- Let someone else take credit for a job you've done.

- Refuse help when you need it or wait until you're in over your head to keep you from drowning.

- Keep doing more and more in the hopes of getting attention and recognition.

- Be afraid of speaking your mind appropriately.

- Let guilt or fear of feeling it dictate what you choose to do or not do.

- Allow yourself to be constantly stressed and believe you can't do anything about it.

- Imagine that you're indispensable because you're not and neither is anyone else in your workplace.

- Automatically pick up someone's slack because you don't want him or her to get into trouble.

- Lose sleep over work or let it take over your life.

Real-life tips for de-nicing at work

A word here about consequences of changing behavior at work versus with friends or family. Because you're paid for what you do, you do have to be a wee bit cautious about how you approach de-nicing yourself. Your employers are not like your friends or family—if your brother doesn't speak to you for a year, so what; if you lose a friend, you'll find another. But the consequences of changing behavior at work are generally more serious. I don't want you to lose your job. If you decide on your own that it's too stressful or doesn't bring out your best qualities, well, good for you. Move on. But until you make the decision that you're out of there, take change slowly.

Try on new behavior gradually; talk to a friendly boss or supervisor about how best to go about standing up for yourself. Let people know that you're trying to be more up front and solicit feedback from people you trust. Go slowly and take baby steps. Find someone outside your job to use as a support, a person who doesn't have a stake in how things go at work or in you acting one way over another. Give yourself time to change and notice how you feel about you: If you're feeling better and better about yourself and have more pride and confidence, you're moving in the right direction, no matter what anyone else says.

Sometimes when you assert yourself at work, people will start to treat you differently. You'll notice some being cold and standoffish and others showing you more respect, including not violating your personal boundaries. It may take them a while if they have a stake in you being Ms. Nice, but give them time to get used to the new you and see how the dust settles.

To do today

If it will stress you out, refuse a request at work.

Meet One of the Nice Girls

Lyla now
Lyla, head librarian at a prestigious university, is fifty-one and has two grown daughters. Well coiffed and expensively

dressed, she's one hundred pounds overweight and has traveled up and down the scale since college. To say she's sick and tired of being fat doesn't begin to describe her disgust and despair. After two nasty divorces, she admits to being "lonelier than lonely" and says she'd love to meet a man, especially to have someone to lean on, but she's also scared out of her mind of being vulnerable again.

So she works—and works. Although she purports to love her job, she frequently spends therapy sessions complaining about her workload and the "never-ending battle to stay on top of things." When pressed, she acknowledges that she thrives on the challenge of providing library patrons with the information they need and that she glows with pleasure each time someone tells her that no one could ever fill her shoes. She's also a much sought after consultant who travels around the country troubleshooting for other university library systems. However, she can't enjoy her accomplishments because she feels guilty when she can't meet requests, agonizes over giving out incorrect information, and ruminates about the advice she gives as a consultant.

Lyla came to therapy, as many of my clients do, through my Quit Fighting with Food workshop. She talks incessantly about her job, as if it's the only thing she has going for her. She regularly misses workshop and individual therapy sessions because she says she has to work or is too exhausted to do anything but go home and crawl into bed. Additionally, she suffers from severe migraines that all but debilitate her for days at a time.

The only thing Lyla loves more than being needed in her job and sleeping is cheesecake, which she orders online and has delivered weekly. She enjoys a special ritual of eating two pieces every Friday night to celebrate that the week is finally over— the first piece is savored right after she walks in the door and the second while she watches mindless TV. Between slices, she eats dinner and maybe a few snacks. Although Lyla understands that she must find better ways to take care of herself, it seems like mission impossible. She joined a health club but doesn't go, makes dates with friends that she often cancels because she's tired, and promises to learn other ways to relax, which never seem to take hold for more than a few weeks. She hates using food to feel better but equally hates the idea of giving it up.

Lyla as a child

Lyla was an only child who lived for the affection of her workaholic, distant father, a lawyer. During his rare moments at home, he was often in his basement office. Even when he was with her, Lyla recalls that he seemed preoccupied, "as if I didn't exist." He was kind to her, but "like a phantom, there but not there." Her mother was always trying to entice Dad to stick around—by making him and Lyla exotic meals from scratch and baking him luscious desserts while she battled to stay thin, dressed beautifully, and kept busy with housework and volunteer activities. She pressured Lyla to be her carbon copy. When Lyla complained about wanting more from her father, her mother would plaster a smile on her face and talk about the need for them to be accepting because he was an "excellent provider and, basically, a good man."

An active child, Lyla was a member of many school clubs and societies. Although her mother made a big deal of her activities, her father gave her very little praise (or criticism). She began gaining weight in college, which was upsetting to her mother who told her, "You'll never find a man if you don't look good." Despite her mother's warnings, she found two husbands and had a daughter with each one, but the men were self-centered and condescending and made Lyla feel terrible about herself. She admits she stayed too long in each marriage and is glad she got out when she did.

De-nicing Lyla

Lyla and I talk a great deal about her work patterns. She admits that work is the only place she feels halfway competent but that she doesn't *really* feel competent there. Or rather, she does and doesn't, describing it like this: "I like the challenge, though it scares me every time I have a request that I won't succeed. When I finally find the right info for someone, I feel good for about twelve seconds, until the next question. It's exhausting." Much of our work centers around her fears of failure and making mistakes. This is a subject we always come back to and that needs to be resolved before she can relax more at work—or maybe even seek a more satisfying job.

She says she's a total failure in the romance department and despairs looking for a partner because she's convinced she'll hook up with another man like her father and exes. When we talk about how she quested after her father's attention and affection, she sometimes sheds a few tears, but then she feels self-pity and stops, sounding like her mother when she shrugs and says, "He did the best he could."

Discussing her Friday night food ritual she laughs bitterly, unable to believe that this is what her life has come to, that its highlight is cheesecake. She describes the taste ("tangy") and texture ("creamy and light"), and I explore what might give her the same feelings, interpreting that she needs some spice and lightness in her life, with which she agrees. She makes a pact with herself to start going out with friends or taking herself to a movie on Friday nights to break her cheesecake jones, but it's hard to drag herself out after an exhausting week. We try other strategies, like scheduling a massage or a facial—even going home and hitting the sack. Nothing works all the time, but she's making inroads and spending less on cheesecake.

What's Next? *In Chapter 7, "Saying What You Mean,"
you'll learn*

- What you're afraid of when you don't speak honestly and from the heart

- What you learned in your family about silence, passivity, assertiveness, and rocking the boat

- How to start using your mouth to speak up rather than eat over your feelings

SEVEN

What Part of "No" Don't You Understand?

Saying What You Mean

There are two major reasons to open your mouth—to speak and to eat. Neither behavior is better than the other. Both are necessary for a pleasurable, productive life and each expresses an inherent, universal human need. The desire to speak your needs and feed your belly are both innate and hardwired into your DNA, as well as shaped by your early experiences with family and culture. Stepping back and observing both activities, anyone can see how clearly distinct they are; other than using the same area of the body, eating and speaking have relatively little in common. So how come nice girls get them confused?

Okay, raise your hand if you . . . have trouble saying what's on your mind most of the time; think hard and long about what you want to say before saying it; worry about sounding mean, unkind, selfish, needy, or demanding; fear offending or hurting someone with your words; feel one thing and say another. These patterns speak volumes about how you see yourself and wish to be seen. After all, how will people know what a charmer you are if you don't use nicespeak?

I'm not suggesting you turn into Ms. Potty Mouth. No one would want to live in a society in which common sense and attempts to commune harmoniously were trampled by being on the tell-it-like-it-is-all-the-time news station. Each of us knows people who blurt out anything that comes to mind whether it offends or not and, if we're smart, we keep as far away from them as possible. I had a client whose mother used to say, "Do you expect me to think every time I open my mouth?" Well, yes, Mom, that's *exactly* what we expect.

But, you nice girls, you've turned nicespeak into an art form! Your speech is so overpeppered with words and phrases like "please," "thank you," "would you mind if," and "I'm sorry" that it's amazing you can cram any other words in between them. You're stuck in some crummy habits, and these can be changed, but not until you understand how they've come about and stolen your honest and authentic voice.

▌**GRAB YOUR THINKING CAP** Do you overuse "please," "thank you," and "I'm sorry" to the point of saying them so often that they've become meaningless? Do you censor your words carefully and try very hard not to offend? Do you hold back saying unkind things, even when people deserve to hear them and you deserve to say them? ▐

You mean silence isn't always golden?

Well, sometimes it is and sometimes it isn't. Reflecting before speaking, holding your tongue, being a good listener, and speaking kindly whenever you can make for excellent communication. However, these verbal skills are only half of what you need in the game of life. The other half is to break a silence and speak up, draw your words from authentic feeling, take care of yourself through what you say even if it hurts someone else's feelings, and use your voice to enhance your life. You already have a terrific set of skills and now need to add another set in order to be complete and in balance. The good news is that these skills are absolutely learnable; the bad news is that you will be extremely uncomfortable developing them. Sorry, there's no other way, so stop thinking about how hard it is to change and gather your courage, optimism, and determination.

One of the reasons we believe silence is golden is because that's what we're told from day one in our culture. Pretty much every society has its equivalent directive to help people keep their traps shut. It's a necessary rule for people living in community, a great lesson, but only a partial one. Rarely do we hear the other half: to speak up when we need to. Because we're told as children to pipe down and are "shushed" to death at home, school, library, and church or synagogue, we think that being silent is preferable to being vocal. Consider what culture teaches us: Don't speak unless you have something important to say, keep your mouth shut unless spoken to, still waters run deep (as if being quiet means you're a deep thinker), hold your tongue, speak softly and carry a big stick, watch your mouth, hush up, shut up, stay mum, and zip your lip. There are oodles of ways to silence us and make us think that there's something wrong with speaking out or sharing what's on our minds.

Now, of course, I wouldn't want to live in a chaotic say-whatever's-on-your-mind society any more than you would. All I'm saying is that there is far more of a cultural push for us to pipe down than for us to pipe up, and that message comes across loud and clear from our earliest days. We're not programmed to enjoy squalling infants, boisterous children, or loud-mouthed adults, so of course we come to believe that silencing ourselves is a good thing for us and everyone else.

Interestingly, females begin life with the gift of gab. Susan Brownmiller in her groundbreaking book *Femininity* maintains that, "From infancy onward little girls excel at verbal skills. . . . Girls begin to talk earlier, are quicker to speak in fluent sentences . . . and have a larger pre-school vocabulary" than boys do.[3] It's curious and profoundly sad how little girls start out so highly verbal and end up being viewed as chatterboxes, shrews, busybodies, or Chatty Cathies who speak only when their cords are pulled.

Suffice it to say that the downward spiral women take—or, more accurate, are thrown into—has to do with both biology and socialization. As discussed previously, the genders are hardwired differently in numerous ways, which was an exceptionally clever and useful approach at the beginning of humankind but is no longer of much value as our species has evolved and gender roles have expanded and blurred. Expectations for boys and girls—and men and women—differ hugely and often are reinforced in opposite directions. Remember, behaviors that are repeated, especially early on, activate neural pathways and make them grow, and behaviors that aren't encouraged die off unless we make a concerted effort to engage in them. In short, women's silence, reticence, and tendency toward sweet talk is due to how our brains have been pruned.

Aren't you going to tell us how our family warped our ability to speak our minds?

Of course I'm going to enlighten you on how family affects your capacity to use your voice to express your needs. The truth is that cultural and gender influences (no matter how strong) can be overridden if you grow up with parents who listen intently (called active listening), validate your ideas and emotions, and encourage you to say what's on your mind. Women who are lucky enough to have parents like this have an operating template that predisposes them to be open, forthright, and direct. For whatever reason, you didn't get this message. Your verbal template is of long-suffering silence, waiting for it to be your turn, offering eternal gratitude to anyone willing to turn an ear your way, swallowing your anger, mincing words, sweet-talking your way out of situations, speaking out of both sides of your mouth, back-pedaling, or saying what you need to in order to survive.

If you're feeling a need to blame yourself, stop now. You didn't choose your family and the communication corner you were backed into. You developed by copying what you heard and adapting to your environment. Nor is it time well spent railing against your parents and how they mistreated your utterances so that you ended up being fluent in nicespeak only. The goal is to be curious about how you developed and understand that while your behaviors were adaptive in the past (for physical and emotional survival), they are now destructive.

Speaking is a by-product of being listened to. Sure, effective parents coo at us, but they also take time to listen to our wails and burbles and respond to them in an encouraging, positive, mirroring, caring tone of voice. They create a kind of duet— sometimes using their voice in tandem with ours, mimicking us, sometimes speaking alone, and other times keeping silent so that we can spout off by ourselves. Their speech and silence and their response to our speech and silence act as guides to communication; their quiet makes space for our voice and their verbal responses reinforce our right to it.

If this sounds like someone else's family, not yours, you're reading the right book. There are many ways that free and open speech can be derailed while we're living under our parents' roof. Maybe there were simply too many children to be adequately heard and addressed. If you have more than a few siblings, even if you had gold standard parents, they may not have had time to hear you out and help you verbalize your inner thoughts and desires. After all, when everyone has to take a turn, and there are many people involved, no one gets the floor very often or for long. Clue: If you can't relinquish the floor once you get it or never really feel heard, you might have grown up around too many mouths and not enough ears.

Maybe your parents were right up front and told you that what you had to say didn't matter or that you were talking through your hat or had a big mouth. Maybe they told you outright to "shut up" or "pipe down" so often that you finally gave up saying anything other than mumbling "please" and "thank you." Perhaps your parents tried to listen but were too exhausted or preoccupied to take in your words and only pretended to hear you. Or maybe they walked out of the room when you began to speak or turned away to start another activity. Either way, you got the message that what came out of your mouth wasn't worth listening to.

You may be wondering what not being listened to and having your words validated has to do with being addicted to nicespeak. Some individuals whose verbal communication skills weren't validated become angry and take every opportunity to vent their anger. We all know people like this, whom we say have a chip on their shoulder. These people rarely have anything nice to say (and, need I remind you, are best kept at a distance).

However, other individuals (like you) learn to limit themselves to saying nice things in the hopes that they will be more acceptable to others' ears than what you really think and feel. After all, it makes sense that folks, especially parents, want to hear good things rather than bad things. So you get their attention and approval by saying cheery, comforting, sweet things. You shower people with praise you don't feel, support them in doing things that aren't necessarily good for them (or you), or say nothing. Your words get shaped around *their* needs, not yours.

One very specific way you learn to speak nicely as a child is when parents or other adults tell you that you shouldn't feel a certain way. You say you're angry at your brother for dismembering Barbie and feeding her body parts to the dog and Mom or Dad chides you with, "Oh, don't say that. You know little Danny didn't mean it." You tell your father that Mom was so mad at you she wouldn't drive you to dance lessons, and he says, "Mom's having a hard time. You should be more patient and understanding of her."

No need to comment on what those remarks do to a fragile, forming psyche. Instead of speaking your feelings or the truth, you learn to go silent or agree with lies. You deny authentic feelings and make sure they're never, ever spoken aloud. After a while, you even forget what the truth is because you've been speaking falsehoods for so long.

Two more scenarios and I'll move off this family stuff. Say you had a parent who was depressed or debilitated in some way. You may have been socialized not to be a burden on her but took enormous pleasure in cheering her up and seeing her smile. So instead of talking about what was really on your mind (being teased in school, failing math, ongoing fights with your twin sister, how your boyfriend broke your heart, etc.), you made sure to share only upbeat, happy thoughts. This worked like a charm: Tell Mom a funny story or say sweet things about her and her face would light up. Pleasing a parent is irresistible to a child but dangerous for healthy emotional growth when every negative thought or feeling has to be squashed out of existence.

On a more benign front, maybe your parents were the two

nicest people on the face of the earth. They never got mad or argued in front of you, had nary a bad word to say about anyone, and blipped every negative into a positive: Rain doesn't ruin picnics but feeds the flowers, going hungry teaches you how to do without or conserve, turning the other cheek makes you a stronger person, speaking badly of someone only shows you in a bad light. If you rarely heard people express negative thoughts and feelings, how could you possibly know how to do this now? Moreover, how would you recognize that such behavior is normal and natural? You wouldn't.

▌**GRAB YOUR THINKING CAP** How did your family shape you to say nice things and keep your real opinions to yourself? ▌

What makes me so tongue-tied that I can't say what I mean?

There are several ways to get tripped up when niceness just rolls off your tongue. You misspeak because you feel guilty, fear hurting other people's feelings, or don't believe you're worthy or deserving. Of course, some of you have limited your vocabulary to nice for all of the above reasons and will have to hunker down and work doubly hard to de-nice yourselves.

You feel guilty

In my *Food and Feelings Workbook* I spend a whole juicy chapter talking about guilt, so if you want to know more about this complex emotion, check it out. For now, let's say that guilt is a feeling that is meant to help you do what you think is right. It taps you on the shoulder when you make mistakes and don't live up to your standards. Of course, these standards need to be reasonable and should be based on the fact that you are and will always be imperfect.

If you live in a perpetual state of guilt and wrong feeling, every word out of your mouth will be directed toward rectifying this situation. If you were brought up to believe that you were born a sinner and should spend the rest of your life seeking salvation, you are on mission impossible. I'm not here to challenge religious teachings that enhance your life, but mindless adherence to principles that fly in the face of good mental health only keep you locked up in Niceville prison. To break out, you need to rethink what you believe spiritually and make some hard choices. Nice girls tend to think in rigid terms of saint and sinner and good and evil, so make sure that your religious beliefs are healthy enough to support the fact that none of us is all good or all bad.

Guilt is appropriate when you've done something wrong, not when you've done something right for you that happens not to suit someone else. Life isn't fair and it never will be. You'll get hurt, I'll get hurt, we'll all get hurt, and guess what?—we'll all live through it. I've said it before and I'll keep saying it: If you hurt someone in the process of taking care of yourself, it's okay. That is my exception to the Golden Rule. So if you're in the habit of yessing people to death because you don't want to feel guilty saying no, you're going to have to start evaluating whether your guilt is appropriate or not. In fact, saying yes when you mean no (because no is right for *you*) is what *should* make you feel guilty. Saying no to take care of yourself shouldn't prompt a guilt trip but should make you proud. Chew on that for a while.

You fear hurting other people's feelings

It isn't possible to write about guilt without touching on the issue of hurt feelings, so you have a little of my thinking on the subject already. If you always try to be nice and balk at speaking your mind because people will feel hurt, you'll have to get over this fear, plain and simple. I understand that you're afraid you'll make them angry at you and that they might reject, humiliate, or abandon you because of it. You're right, they might. But now that you're a grown-up and can stand on your own two feet, you no longer need to be beholden to or afraid of them. If you need additional help on giving yourself permission to hurt others' feelings, you'll find more information in Chapter 9, "People Pleasing."

Naturally, if you're going to get emotionally or physically whacked around because you share your feelings, you will have to take this whole process a bit slower. Until you're safe, you'll need to be careful about what you say. Remember, verbal harangues can sometimes cross over into physical abuse. If you regularly fear abuse and are not in counseling, call someone immediately. I mean it. Keep making calls until you find someone who can help. Plus, if you're in physical danger, get out or start making plans to leave as soon as possible.

Okay, back to those of you who are only in perceived danger when you think about saying what you mean. So what if the president of the garden club is ticked at you for declining to lead another house tour? Will you starve, go naked, lose the roof over your head? No? Then forget about her. So what if your boss insists you stay late even though he knows you have Knicks tickets to celebrate your anniversary? Too bad. If he's going to fire you for that, you've been in the wrong job for too long. Often nice girls actually choose circumstances that keep them mum by surrounding themselves with family, friends, and colleagues who reinforce their niceness and silence. If you're stuck in such a situation, start speaking up and work on getting out.

You don't believe you're worthy or deserving
It's hard to voice true feelings and advocate for yourself when you don't believe you're of much value. People who feel like

second-class citizens tend to accept whatever they get and avoid reaching out for more. Maybe you're convinced that you deserve to have people mistreat you or that your destiny is to spend your life taking care of others and not yourself. Perhaps you have some misguided belief that folks will magically do right by you even if you don't tell them what right is and they've been doing you wrong all along. That belief is wishful, childlike thinking, not adult assessment and communication. Or you might think that if you keep quiet, people won't be offended and will like you more.

Being invisible and devaluing yourself is a strategy you learned in childhood to get you through the tough times, but no one is going to think much of you now unless you start to value yourself. And what better way to let people know how thrilled you are to be little ole you than to be verbal about your needs and desires. If you don't like to rock the boat, what kind of vessel are you floating around in? Certainly not one that's strong and well crafted and can survive rough seas. Building yourself up by speaking up and saying what you mean not only reinforces your value in your own eyes but also encourages people to treat you respectfully.

▌ GRAB YOUR THINKING CAP Do you avoid saying what you mean because if you did, you'd feel guilty? Because you're afraid of hurting people's feelings? Because you don't think enough of yourself to take good care of you? ▌

What happens if people don't like me when I say what I really mean?

I don't know. You tell me what will happen. Or, rather, what you *fear* will happen. Will some catastrophe befall you . . . or will you merely be uncomfortable as hell for a little while? The truth is that if people withdraw love, you'll find others to love you. If they try to hurt you emotionally or physically, in most cases you can fight back or walk away from them. If they try to make you feel bad about being forthright, you can remind yourself that no one who really cares about you would want you to be dishonest and turn against yourself. If they abandon you, you'll find others to help you and learn to stand on your own two feet by developing and drawing from inner resources.

One of the biggest problems you create by avoiding confrontation, fudging the truth, making nice with words, and allowing yourself to be silenced is that you lose respect for yourself, which leads to feeling ashamed. When you stand up for yourself, you might be frightened, but the end product is that—no matter what happens—you will always have the pride of having spoken out on your own behalf. Nothing can replace that feeling—no amount of false love or approval from someone else, no amount of security or money, no external prize you believe you'll win by compromising your values, opinions, desires, and beliefs. Believe me, nothing feels as good as honest and proud.

Is there a link between stuffing my feelings and stuffing my face?

Need you ask? Of *course* there's a link and an important one. Remember I said in the beginning of this chapter that there are two reasons to open your mouth—to eat and to speak? Well, you're having a bit of a problem keeping them straight. We might say that you overeat because you underspeak or that you eat over your feelings. When you share feelings appropriately, effectively, and in a timely manner, believing that you have the right to do so and that what you say has a profound effect in shaping your life, voicing your opinions becomes a positive aspect of self. When you worry constantly about offending, saying the wrong thing, or not being understood or heard, speaking up becomes a burden and causes tremendous anxiety.

By swallowing your feelings, you end up mired in them. They grow larger and create more and more distress. Stress brings you nearer to the breaking point and keeps inching you closer and closer to finding something to help you chill out. That that something is food is no news to you. Not only do you look to food for comfort, but because it gives your mouth something to do rather than speak, eating feels right. Think about it. If you weren't stuffing yourself silly, you might be saying something that could hurt someone or letting her know that she's hurt you. Better to keep that mouth occupied, so it doesn't run off and get you in trouble.

NO MORE NICE GIRL MANIFESTO FOR SAYING WHAT YOU MEAN

DO

- Think long and hard before responding to requests and demands.

- Stop feeling guilty when you say no, or ride out the guilt.

- Risk not getting approval if you need to confront or challenge someone.

- Recognize that it's not your job to make everyone else feel better.

- Acknowledge that you're allowed to be imperfect and make mistakes.

- Let people know in an appropriate way, in the moment or after the fact, when they've hurt you.

- Keep track of what you're feeling so that you can speak the truth about what's going on inside you.

- Give yourself time to understand what you *really* think before putting emotions into words.

- Learn to tolerate feeling uncomfortable when you've been honest and direct and someone is upset (because nine out of ten times he or she will get over it).

- Realize that it's far better to feel good about yourself for being honest than bad about yourself for lying to avoid conflict.

- Understand that self-trust develops from decisions that make you proud.

- Recognize that no one (except sadists) enjoys hurting someone's feelings, but that healthy people do it to take care of themselves.

- Recognize that you have every right to say what is on your mind in an appropriate, timely manner no matter what anyone tells you.

DON'T

- Automatically say yes because you think it's expected or you'll feel guilty saying no.

- Be afraid of speaking your mind appropriately.

- Let guilt or fear of experiencing it dictate what you choose to do or not do.

- Lie to yourself or you'll end up not knowing what you really feel.

- Think that people can't tolerate or get over hurt feelings, because they can.

- Avoid conflict because it makes you or someone else uncomfortable.

- Allow others to mistreat you without speaking up about how it feels.

- Silently tolerate ongoing physical, sexual, or verbal abuse—ever.

- Stew in silence, deny your feelings, or let them build until you're ready to explode.

- Act passive-aggressively (let negative feelings out in a vague, indirect way that you don't have to be accountable for) because it's easier than being direct.

- Let people decide for you what's okay and not okay for you to say.

- Assume that people know how you feel if you don't tell them.

- Allow yourself to become a scapegoat or whipping girl without protesting immediately.

- Assume that other people can't handle your authentic feelings.

One last word about saying what you mean. You can't speak the truth if you don't know what *your* truth is. If you continually deny your feelings and let people tell you what you should and shouldn't feel, you'll definitely end up confused. If people (friends, family, coworkers) constantly invalidate your feelings and inhibit you from speaking freely, slowly wean yourself away from them. Search often and deeply for what is authentic in you and gradually start putting it out into the world. Try keeping a feelings journal or speaking to yourself in front of a mirror. Finding your voice is a scary process, for sure, but it can't be any scarier than living a lie of a life based on a foundation of fear. The truth, *your* truth, will set you free.

To do today

Speak honestly in a situation where you usually lie or speak up in one in which you're generally silent.

Meet One of the Nice Girls

Alison now

You can tell just by meeting Alison that she's a good girl, or at least tries to be. She has a sweet smile, which she flashes shyly in our first session as she tells me in a soft voice that she's thrilled to meet me. Single and twenty-six, she's a paralegal and talks vaguely of someday going to law school. She lives with her parents and, after several sessions, volunteers that she thinks about moving out, but every time she brings up the subject, her parents "go berserk," so she drops it. Her friends think she should find her own place, but her fiancé keeps pressing her to continue living at home to save money until they get married.

Alison admits that she's terrible at speaking her mind and terrified of conflict. It's difficult for her to say *anything* unkind about her parents, but she ventures that it's "annoying" that her mother is always telling her what to do and that her father basically goes along with whatever her mother wants. Alison is proud that she's done well in school and has made something of herself, but she remains torn about declaring independence.

Although Alison doesn't have a weight problem, she does have eating issues. She goes on eating binges and purges, which she can barely speak about. She tells me she's had an eating disorder since her teens but that no one—not even her fiancé—knows about it. "I'd rather die than have anyone find out," she whispers. When she finally makes the connection between not speaking her mind and using her mouth to binge and purge, she's so startled tears flood her eyes. She cries even harder when I tell her this is the first time I've seen and heard her share a deeply felt, authentic feeling.

When asked to give me examples of not speaking her mind, she offers the following: "Oh, you now, I'm always willing to stay late at work or go get one of the lawyers lunch even though it's not part of my job description and makes me get behind." She often makes faces after comments like this, as if her expression is broadcasting emotions her mouth dare not speak. Sadly, she acknowledges that she usually lets her fiancé make most of the decisions whether she agrees with him or not, but is quick to add that, "He's a lot smarter than I am, so it only makes sense." When she gives me that shy smile, I can see a hint of sadness behind her pearly whites and pink lipstick.

Alison as a child

Alison's parents are very religious and the family goes back three generations in the community. Her older brother is a missionary in Africa and her youngest brother plans to study pastoral counseling. To her recollection, neither of them ever talked about wanting to do anything else. Her mother is what she calls "a woman of good works" and her father, a middle manager in a local furniture company, is a church deacon. Alison was never encouraged to think or speak for herself. Her mother frequently admonished, "Oh, don't say that," "You can't mean that," or "You have to learn to push bad thoughts out of your mind if you want to ascend to heaven," while her father lectured her about what "nice girls" did and did not do. Both parents believe in heaven and hell, take the Bible literally, and never allowed their children to miss Sunday school or church services.

Alison received A's in conduct in school and was often teacher's pet. Under her high school yearbook photo (she smiles wistfully when she shows it to me) is written, "Would that everyone were as easygoing and sweet as Alison. Her smile will take her far." There is a part of her that understands that she will not go anywhere or overcome her bingeing and purging problems until she stops being so easygoing, sweet, and smiley faced.

De-nicing Alison

This is one of those cases where I do most of the work in what's called the transference (her reacting to me with the same feelings and behaviors she did to significant people in her childhood—her parents). Because Alison wants so badly to please me (along with everyone else she meets), I encourage her to speak up and let me know when I'm doing something that hurts or puzzles her. It takes a long time, but eventually she learns to say what's on her mind (though often not until three or four sessions after the occurrence). She's amazed that I actually want her to assert herself and that I don't get upset or angry when she does.

Next we zero in on her speaking up with friends she trusts and work our way down the line to folks at work, her fiancé, and her parents. The work is arduous and generally after Alison takes a risk and says her piece, we spend the next few sessions dissecting what happened. Simultaneously, we talk about her food binges and purges and what they mean to her, when they occur, why she continues these behaviors, and what strategies she can use to prevent them. Although there's a general reduction in disordered eating, she can't go for more than a week without returning to food or body abuse. I know she's at least on her way when one day she comes into session saying (without smiling), "I think I need to grow up rather than throw up."

What's Next? *In Chapter 8, "Overcoming Perfectionism," you'll learn*

- Why you feel a need to be perfect and what you fear about being imperfect

- How shame, helplessness, and anxiety underlie your need for perfectionism

- How to start enjoying being imperfect and accepting mistakes and failure

EIGHT

Can I Be Perfectly Imperfect?

Overcoming Perfectionism

I f you're a perfectionist—and my hunch is that most of you sport this label—you probably know it, but for any of you who aren't quite certain, here are the telltale signs. Doing something slapdash is a no-no; you can't leave well enough alone; you think mediocrity is a cardinal sin; you believe that if something isn't completely right, it must be completely wrong; people are always telling you to slow down and take it easy; you fear that others won't do as good a job as you do and find delegating as painful as having a tooth extracted; you're driven by fear of failure and of making mistakes; you don't distinguish between behaviors you'd like to do exceptionally well and those you can afford to do half-assed because of time, energy, skill, talent, other commitments, resources, etc.

Okay, now, raise your hand if you recognize yourself. Oh, I see some of you out there with both hands raised. And a few of you have taken off your shoes and are waving your feet as well. In case there are still a handful of you who aren't sure if you're a perfectionist, let me explain what perfectionism is not. It isn't wanting to do certain things to the best of your ability. It's not having dreams and goals toward which you work feverishly. Nor is it a desire to excel and reach the top. *Perfectionism means feeling an intense, driving inner (often unconscious) pressure to do everything right or well no matter whether you harm yourself in the process.* The operant words here are "pressure," "everything," and "harm yourself." Perfectionism is part obsession—your mind sinks its teeth into desire and won't let it go—and part compulsion—your body then runs off to take action to put desire into play.

With perfectionism, objective analysis and thoughtful judgment fly out the window. You don't stop and think: *Do I have time for this? Could I use some help? What would happen if I stopped now and left things as is? What would happen if I chucked the whole shebang and got a pedicure? How does what I'm doing add to or detract from the quality of my life? Is there something other than obvious desire that's pressing me onward, something more sinister and more compelling and complex?* Being in the grip of perfectionism is similar to the feeling that strikes you when you simply *have to* finish eating something even though you're close to upchucking. The behavior makes no sense. Nevertheless, you do it because if you don't, you'll be (or fear you'll be) intensely distressed.

Because of your ongoing quest to be all things to all people, never disappoint, and always do everything to a tee, there's a good chance that your lips have difficulty shaping no. Oddly, yes just rolls off your tongue. To many nice girls, saying no to requests and demands is impossible because it implies that they're not good enough, are too weak or lazy or inadequate or, worse, are selfish and want to do something for themselves rather than somebody else. No matter how many times you're told that striving for perfection is a fruitless, thankless endeavor, your automatic pilot takes over and you shoot for the stars.

The two main problems with perfectionism are that it feels so darned satisfying and that it's highly prized and rewarded. In a society whose excesses have excess and that willfully turns a blind eye to dysfunctional imbalance and disregulation, perfectionism is often viewed as a very fine thing indeed. Go the extra mile, do it 'til it hurts, sacrifice, more is better, no pain no gain. Once again, culture plays its part in spinning an unhealthy behavior into a near divine attribute.

Exactly how does this happen? Well, first off, think about school and the struggle to compete, achieve, try your hardest, and excel. Consider the supreme honor of being school valedictorian, becoming a member of the honor society, getting into an Ivy League college. Why shouldn't it be okay to do well in some subjects and not others? What's wrong with doing a stellar job in math and a so-so one in French, in acing art and barely getting by in biology? We're unique individuals, not programmed machines. Most educational systems in this country encourage competition and use shame as a motivator, that is, if you don't do well you're either not trying hard enough or don't have what it takes. So we learn to push ourselves beyond healthy endurance and sometimes we succeed (reinforcing perfectionism) and sometimes we don't.

Need I mention sports and other kinds of competition in the form of after-school clubs and activities—dance class, debate club, swimming lessons, Little League, kung fu, Junior League? All this running around from club to class to sports gives kids the impression that they have to do it all and do it all well. These activities are fine in and of themselves, but they lend credence to the erroneous belief *that we have to do and be good at everything*. We can't play softball for the sheer exhilaration of being out in the sunshine with friends whacking the ball around or enjoy the pure pleasure of picking our way through a melody on grandma's old, out-of-tune piano. No, we have to have lessons and the right teacher and practice, practice, practice.

Then there's religion, which encourages us to have only pure thoughts and do only good deeds. Need I remind you of the Ten Commandments? I personally think there needs to be an expanded set of commandments that are not quite so dictatorial and encourage us to think critically for ourselves and stay in balance. Yes, working hard, taking care of others, and trying to be kind and generous are admirable traits (along with not coveting your neighbor's spouse), but not to the exclusion of all others. Where do we receive adequate spiritual guidance to put ourselves first and to do unto *ourselves* as we would do to others? Even thinking this way may feel like blasphemy.

In general, the more deeply steeped you are in religious precepts or the more ingrained your training, the more you may feel the need to hold on to the nice parts of you and discard the rest for fear of not living up to spiritual ideals. Being nice exclusively is a wistful ideal, but not possible. Humans have imperfections and the model of trying to be perfect is not a healthy one. If you're offended by my challenging religious principles, skip this chapter and go on to the next. If you can tolerate the challenge, you have a better chance of overcoming perfectionism and shucking the problems you have with being overly nice and overly attached to food.

▌ GRAB YOUR THINKING CAP How have your educational experiences shaped your need to be perfect? How have competitive activities contributed to your need to excel beyond excellence? How has your religious upbringing or training reinforced
the concept of not sinning, being good, nice, and living up to
unattainable ideals? ▐

What about my upbringing and perfectionism?

Our upbringing is a major factor in determining whether or
not we turn into perfectionists. As with psychiatric and substance disorders, perfectionism tends to run in families. If you
have one parent who's a perfectionist and one who isn't, you
have a fighting chance. If both parents are so inclined, I'd be
surprised if you were able to escape the *p* word. Of course,
what our parents model about the pursuit of excellence is only
one element molding us into poster children for the unflawed.
But it is a key influence.

Here's how it happens. We see Dad or Mom working late,
skipping meals and family events in order to feverishly climb
a career ladder. We watch them clean obsessively or practically kill themselves whipping the garden into shape. Maybe
they refuse to have guests unless the house is in order top to
bottom, push themselves to overachieve at sports and supposed leisure activities, have to be the perfect hosts and never
let guests lift a finger, or wouldn't dream of leaving the house
without looking like Ms. or Mr. America. Often their energy
goes into chiseling an ideal body or devising a rigid diet plan
that will magically make them svelte and slim.

Dirty laundry and messy rooms aren't tolerated. How you
and they look is a big deal and how things appear to the outside
world overshadows how things feel in your heart. They care
what the neighbors think, don't want to embarrass themselves,

hate to let anyone down, stay busy until they get sick or over-come with exhaustion. Being selfish is the worst thing anyone could possibly be. Their ideals are impossible to achieve, but that doesn't stop Mom or Dad from trying. And their pressure on you to conform and excel, even when it's patently obvious to everyone else that it's not in your best interest, is relentless.

It's this combination of modeling perfection and expecting it of you that nails shut your perfect coffin. You share their belief that one person should never disappoint another, so how could you ever dream of not doing what they tell you or not striv-ing to meet their lofty standards? Sometimes parents don't even need to say a word about what they expect of you; it's in their every glance. More than that, it's the unstated family message that perfection is expected and nothing less will be tolerated and how terribly disappointed they'll be if you don't measure up.

To be fair, most parents are completely clueless that they're ruining their children's chances for happiness by placing un-reasonable demands on themselves and their progeny. Instead, they're doing what their parents did, or are simply trying to be helpful and do right by you. They generally have no idea what unfair and undue pressure can do—because they're so out of touch with their own feelings and out of balance in their own lives. Maybe they surround themselves with people exactly like themselves. They certainly get reinforced by our culture. Mostly, they can't imagine being any other way or that there even is another way to be.

However, the drive behind perfection is more complex and subtle than parental modeling and expectations. If there was a tremendous amount of dysfunction and shame-based activity in your house growing up, perfection becomes its antidote. If things look good from the outside, no one will suspect Dad's drinking, Mom's depression, Grandpa's Peeping Tom episodes, or Grandma's shoplifting excursions. If emotional, sexual, or physical abuse is occurring and it's not getting addressed, living a cover story of perfection conceals it. Sadly, just by putting their energy into making life appear so, people can convince themselves that all's right with the world when it isn't.

In this way, perfectionism is a direct reaction to being raised in a shame-based family. Then there's the hope that if you're a good little girl, Mommy won't throw things and Daddy won't stay out all night or get arrested again. *We try to manage situations that are not of our making and over which we have basically no control by being good* because most of us are raised to think that good things happen to good people and bad things happen to bad people. Not so, not so at all. It stands to reason that if being good sometimes calms down Mom or Dad, then being good all the time (that is, perfect) will win the day. You come to believe that if only you can keep up your grades, maintain a spotless room, not fight with your siblings, and do all your chores just right, nothing bad will happen.

When something bad does happen (and it *always* does), you think it's your fault and redouble your efforts rather than understand that your impact as a child on the behavior of your parents or relatives is slim to none. That they're triggered by their own internal impulses is beyond your ability to comprehend, especially when they blame you for their actions and make you feel responsible for their acting badly. As a child you believe they are right and you are wrong. Unfortunately, you build your life around the belief that you can fix other people and the world all by yourself if you only keep trying and trying and never give up. It's the worst kind of rat race, the most lonely treadmill, the saddest example of a dog chasing its tail.

■ **GRAB YOUR THINKING CAP** What behaviors and attitudes did your parents model that have turned you into a perfectionist? In what ways did they interact with you that made you feel you had to be perfect? Do you see how perfectionism is really about trying to avoid shame? ▌

What about all the miserable feelings that plague me when I don't live up to my expectations?

You really are your own worst enemy. It's not bad enough that you race around fielding unreasonable requests, keeping outrageous commitments, propping up fragile egos, and fulfilling everyone's wildest dreams—and still feel inadequate—but you're afflicted with a host of other painful emotions. When you say no, even for very good reason, you feel terribly guilty and have difficulty shaking the feeling. Even proffering the most insignificant refusal can leave you brooding for days on end. No matter how often you apologize, or how frequently your apologies are accepted, you can't stop feeling that you should be immediately sentenced to death by hanging.

You couldn't take your mother to the doctor because you were watching your daughter in her school play or couldn't get to the play in time because you had to rush your mother to the emergency room. You didn't manage to do all sixty-seven things you promised to do in a day and accomplished only forty-three, so you want to crawl under a rock or beat your head with a spatula. No matter how much you do, you feel guilty all the time because there's always more to do. Or if not more, you could have done what you did a whole heck of a lot better.

Most of your activity is due to fear of disappointing others (as if no one in their life has ever been let down before). You think they can't bear it and will emulsify on the spot. You think about the terrible life they've had and don't want to cause any more pain. Or you recognize how they've never known disappointment and you can't stand the idea of being the first not to be there for them. You (wrongly) believe that other people get as bent out of shape when they're disappointed as you do or that they'll never forgive you for taking care of you instead of them.

Some of these ideas are only in your head and some of them are true. There are people who make a big fuss about petty disappointments, who take the slightest hint of rejection as the kiss of death, and who hold a grudge forever. Somehow you surround yourself with these kinds of people as well as those who can't or won't do much for themselves, who need constant reassurance and bolstering, and who see you as the Messiah or, at least, their personal savior. You'd rather be run over by a bus than dash their hopes and dreams.

When you're not feeling guilty or living in terror of disappointing or hurting someone, you're miserable over your own inadequacy. You can't believe you had such high hopes for yourself; with all your talent and energy, how can you fall so short of your goals? You know it's completely unrealistic, but somewhere in your heart you believe you can save the world, or at least most of the people in it. You're constantly measuring yourself against other people or against your ideal self who is a combination of the Energizer Bunny, Superwoman, and Mother Teresa. Your sense of inadequacy is oppressive and overwhelming, and makes you stressed and depressed. What a disappointment you are to yourself!

One odd feeling that crops up occasionally—and is sure to make you uncomfortable enough to head for the leftover lasagna—is resentment. There you are rolling merrily along and suddenly it rears up out of nowhere. You see yourself clearly for a brief moment doing everything for everyone and never spending time taking care of yourself and suddenly you're

Rambo in heels. Why can't people recognize how much you do for them? Why won't they cut you some slack? Why can't they do more for themselves and even do something for you once in a while? You're intensely uncomfortable with this kind of negative feeling and would far prefer feeling guilty and inadequate, emotions that are familiar, so you push the emotions aside or tell yourself you're a bad person for experiencing them—or eat.

This is all very depressing, so is there a way out?

Glad you asked. Of course, there's a way out. Here are tried and true ways you can de-perfect you.

Lower your expectations of yourself

Take an objective look at what you expect of yourself and decide if it's rational, reasonable, and healthy. Check out how much other healthy people do and find out how they deal with letting go, being mediocre, and not working so hard they make themselves sick. Make a list of areas in which you want to keep expectations high (say, being a good parent), those in which you could do a mediocre job (like house cleaning or volunteering in your community), and those in which you can afford to really slack off (mothering people at work, being everyone's best friend). Once your expectations are more realistic, you won't feel so pressured.

Start to accept mistakes and failure

No one likes to do poorly or fail, but some people really don't care all that much about succeeding. They figure that some endeavors aren't worth the energy of giving it their all and that they can do a slapdash job and move on to what they enjoy. They also know the world won't end if they fail. Instead, they expect that they'll learn from things going wrong and that they might be better off in the long run. Shame doesn't overwhelm them, especially when they discuss their shortcomings rather than keep them secret because they know that sharing de-powers shame.

Embrace and enjoy human imperfection

Rather than expect to be perfect, healthy people expect to be imperfect—and they always succeed! They laugh at their goofs and gaffs and don't go out of their way to hush them up. Understanding that everyone makes mistakes, they actually enjoy the flaws of being human. Because they don't have an attachment to perfection, they don't take life so seriously and have a lot more fun. When life is an adventure, there's less room for going morose when things don't work out. Moreover, they know how to get the best mileage out of misadventures, like what terrific stories they'll make down the line.

Ask less from yourself and more from others

Get off your high horse and ask for help. No one really likes martyrs or people who do everything so terrifically and perfectly themselves that they don't need assistance once in a while. An I'll-do-it-myself attitude makes other people feel superfluous and inadequate. People love to feel needed and to be considered supportive and helpful. Make yourself approachable so that folks aren't terrified to offer help because you'll start screaming that you're fine or that you can handle things when you obviously can't. No one is trying to undermine your self-esteem or your independence. Here's a shocker: They like you a lot, enough to want to be helpful.

Avoid all-or-nothing thinking

When you think in extreme either-or terms, you set yourself up for misery, as in if you don't do something perfectly, you're a failure. Hello, how could this be true? If you run for president of the United States and lose but are a senator for twenty-three years, you're a failure? Come on, now. Where does this kind of craziness come from? Measure success in increments and think of achievements on a continuum. Please, scale down your grandiosity. Instead of whining that you didn't do something completely right, think of the fact that you came pretty close. Instead of looking at what you did poorly, focus on what you did well. Remember fractions: one-half, one-quarter, three-quarters, etc.

Don't measure yourself against others

We all start out in a different place in life with diverse genes and dissimilar upbringings. Some people have many talents, others have one amazing one. Most of us are average. Competition is fine as long as you don't put yourself down for not measuring up. Think in terms of making progress from where you were, not comparing yourself to where someone else is. Maybe you started farther back than she did, maybe you had stumbling blocks along the way that she didn't, maybe she's making herself sick being so damed good at what she does.

Learn how to turn off guilt and fear

When you slip into feeling guilty or inadequate or fear disappointing or hurting someone, catch yourself and boycott the feeling. Although I spend the bulk of my professional life nudging people to explore and experience most feelings, some emotions are unproductive and have no place in a healthy life. Unwarranted guilt, fear, and inadequacy are three emotions it's time to wave good-bye to. They won't disappear right away; you'll have to keep shooing them out the door. The more often you allow yourself to wallow in them, the longer they'll stick around.

However, if you experience resentment, pay heed. Maybe it means you're feeling undervalued, which, in turn, might indicate that you either need to do less or ask for more appreciation. Resentment might be pushing you toward reality and health, so don't knock it until you understand what you're feeling.

How does wanting to be perfect make me such an imperfect eater?

One obvious way that perfectionism drives you to overeat is that you use food to cope with stress. Is there anyone out there who doesn't find perfectionism stressful? Here's the progression: The harder you work to be perfect, the more overwhelmed you feel, and the more overwhelmed you feel, the more you want to eat. You eat to slow down, chill out, make time for yourself, recharge your battery, nourish your body, reward yourself, and feel like a human being. Of course, you could do all these things without food, but you don't know how to do that yet.

Perfectionism works in two other ways regarding food. Not surprising, you may want to be a perfect eater, always to eat nutritiously, within a certain calorie range by balancing food groups and eschewing fat, nonorganics, and anything that isn't wholesome. So what happens? Can you stick to your ideal diet? Of course not. Sooner or later (usually sooner) you're bound to have rebound eating, that is, cravings for forbidden foods. These desires are part mental from psychic deprivation and part physiological because you're not choosing from a wide enough range of nutrients and your body wants to be in balance.

The other way that perfectionism impacts eating is that all of us need to have somewhere to make a mess, and your (unconsciously) chosen area is food. No one can keep herself on a tight leash all the time, and the place you break completely free is eating. We could say that overeating makes you human and is trying to drive a point home to you: Cut out all that perfectionism. If you weren't so gung-ho on doing right all the time, you wouldn't have to balance yourself out by "doing wrong" with food. In a way, nature will out even if it has to knock some sense into you in ways you deem unkind.

There's more. Striving for perfection is another way of saying that you don't know when enough is enough, right? Instead of consciously deciding to stop doing, you arrive at "enough" when you hit a wall, reach exhaustion, or there's nothing left to accomplish because you've done it all! Like a blind person feeling her way through life, you rely on external cues to find your way to sufficiency rather than respond to an innate sense of adequacy and doneness.

You keep on saying yes while waiting to feel good, satisfied, full, or complete, but that never happens because there's generally more that can be done—chores or actions, people to help, goals to reach, food to eat, etc. The fact is enough is not some predestined endpoint but comes from a self-determined sense of satisfaction and acceptance—an intuitive feeling of okayness, adequacy, and completion—that resonates within you as a yes (and should come out of your mouth as "no more"). Enough makes itself felt internally and should cause you to say *"basta"* no matter what anyone else thinks, says, or does.

Striving for perfection and not knowing when to cry uncle is eerily similar to not knowing when to stop eating. You keep on chewing and swallowing and stop only when you run out of money, time, or food, not because you have a feeling of fullness and satiation. Perfectionism and overeating are both manifestations of self-regulation difficulties and a kind of tone deafness to sufficiency.

▋ **GRAB YOUR THINKING CAP** Which feelings drive you to eat? Fear of disappointing people? Guilt? Inadequacy? Harboring resentment? All of the above? Do you understand how problems with self-regulation drive both perfectionism and eating problems? ▋

NO MORE NICE GIRL MANIFESTO FOR PERFECTION

DO

- Look for progress, not perfection.

- Laugh at and learn from your mistakes.

- Accept failure as proof of your humanity.

- Share your mistakes and failures with other people in order to de-power them.

- Cultivate curiosity and self-compassion when things go wrong for you.

- Toss out the idea that you can be all things to all people.

- Notice that healthy people get over you occasionally disappointing them.

- Keep away from people who are a drain on your energy.

- Refuse to overdo because someone else is underdoing.

- Remind people that you're not perfect and never expect to be.

- Decide what you want to be excellent, mediocre, or poor at—and stick to your list.

- Think in incremental terms and realize that the opposite of success is not failure.

- Tell people when their expectations are unreasonable and refuse unrealistic demands.

- Ask people for help and accept it graciously when they offer it.

- Enjoy imperfection!

DON'T

- Let other people guilt-trip you into doing things that are unreasonable.

- Wallow in guilt, resentment, inadequacy, or fear of disappointing or hurting others.

- Let other people set expectations for you.

- Hide your failures and mistakes and get stuck in shame.

- Say no to help if you need it.

- Focus on achievement over being engaged in the moment.

- Expect other people to be perfect.

- Allow yourself to become a martyr or a victim.

- Use food to comfort yourself when you don't reach your goals.

- Ignore body signals that tell you when you're tired, sick, or have done too much.

Okay, here's what I think is going to happen to all you perfectionists: You're going to try to do all of the above perfectly. No, no, no. Loosen up. Perfection is a hard trait to let go of and it's going to take a lot of practice and discomfort on your part to think and act like a human being, not a goddess. You'll do well for a while, then go on a perfection jag. Sometimes you'll think clearly about self-expectations and sometimes you'll get all twisted up again in old, familiar idealistic attitudes. You won't progress in a straight line, that I can promise you. Cheer yourself on for every positive and negative step. That way you cover all the bases. Your new goal should be aspiring to be an actual human being, not a mythical ideal.

To do today

Make a mistake and laugh at it or tell someone about it in a humorous way.

Meet One of the Nice Girls

Faith now

Faith, thirty-seven, came into our first session bubbling with joy and gratitude for her happy, perfect life. She's worked her way up as a decorator to having a few well-paying clients, loves her orthopedic surgeon husband, and has four adorable (I saw pictures!) children, toddler through teens. Then, a few sessions down the road, she confessed that her life isn't really perfect but that it would be if only she could stop struggling with food and her body, which she dislikes intensely. Like most people, she classifies food as "good" or "bad," and can't stay on a diet without sneaking "really bad stuff and then feeling like I want to kill myself." She hates being fat (she's forty-five pounds overweight) and unable to fit into her expensive, well-tailored clothes, but is almost as miserable when she's thinner and starving herself. She's finally decided she can't stay on such a crazy merry-go-round and is ready to "overcome my eating issues" by learning to eat "normally."

One of Faith's major difficulties is making decisions. Unfortunately, her husband is the same way. Their old Lexus actually died on the road (with the entire family in it) because they couldn't settle on what kind of new car to buy. They worry about everything—how making wrong decisions will affect them, their kids, their finances, and their future—then second-guess themselves as soon as a decision is made. Another of Faith's problems is distress about people seeing her flaws. She's obsessive about keeping a clean house and loves to entertain friends and her husband's colleagues with lavish dinner parties. On the other hand, she always plays down achievements and once told a friend that a dress costing $335 was a find in a thrift shop!

Faith knows that perfection is a huge issue for her, but she's uncomfortable doing things only so-so and not micromanaging every corner of her life. She explains that the reason she does so well as a decorator is her obsessive attention to detail and the fact that she won't stop searching for exactly what she's looking for until she finds it. She insists that perfectionism is what makes her business so successful. Moreover, she frequently pushes me for a guarantee that therapy will straighten out her eating problems and land her at a comfortable, healthy weight she can maintain for life. Mostly she "hates that I can't overcome this one thing that's so wrong with me, 'cause if I did, my life really would be perfect!"

Faith as a child

The family in which Faith grew up was much like her current one. Financial success and material goods were highly prized and spending money for show was strongly encouraged. Although she now sees that her parents had "little to say to each other," from the outside, the family—Faith and two brothers—looked ideal. No one (not even the boys!) was allowed to get dirty and everyone had to clean up messes on the spot. Each child had chores to complete and Faith's parents were diligent inspectors. If she left her closet a mess to go out and play, her mother would search the neighborhood to find her and tell her (quietly but firmly) that she had to come home and straighten up before she could go out again.

Looking back, Faith recognizes that all along she sensed an undercurrent of anxiety in her parents but couldn't understand where it came from. They were both in excellent health, finances were no problem, and they seemed to have lots of friends and a pretty darned good life. She now realizes that they were afraid of something happening to destroy their picture-perfect world and transferred their anxiety onto their children. One of her brothers has a personality similar to hers and is an overachiever. The other one is "a mess, but no one ever talks about him and, instead, pretends he doesn't exist." Faith admits that she easily could be like her mess of a brother if she ever stops being so hypervigilant.

De-nicing Faith

Perfection is a theme of therapy, actually, *the* theme. Faith always has a check in hand when she arrives exactly on time. She watches the clock faithfully so she won't run a minute over and throws herself heart and soul into examining why she does "this awful stuff to my body and why I hate it so much." She takes notes compulsively in session and is reluctant to leave without my giving her some kind of homework, which, of course, she always completes.

Because Faith is so focused on eating problems, we spend a part of every session talking about them. Slowly she begins to understand that the only place she allows herself to make a mess is with food and that she keeps making a mess (overeating) and cleaning it up (feeling badly) compulsively. She also recognizes that she doesn't really know what she's afraid of if she and her life aren't perfect, but she's beginning slowly to let go of her ideas about control and entertain ones of what it might be like just to be herself. This is very painful work and the anxiety generated about finding out who she really is makes her want to jump out of her skin. Recently she had an insight that her parents are empty vessels internally/emotionally and she fears maybe she is too, making her wonder if that's what she's scared of discovering. The truth is that clients like Faith (who, ironically, has so little in herself) are wonderful to work with because their perfectionism drives them to find answers—and they often succeed.

What's Next? *In Chapter 9, "People Pleasing," you'll learn*

- Why you try so hard to earn folks' approval

- Where the desire to please people comes from

- How stopping people pleasing will help curb emotional eating

NINE

Please Please Me, Oh Yeah!

People Pleasing

Once upon a time you were a tiny organism who pleased no one but herself. You cried when you felt like it, ate when you were hungry and were offered sustenance, slept when you were tired, soiled your diapers, screamed when you wanted to be picked up, and generally wreaked havoc on the needs and schedules of everyone around you. You didn't give a hoot about anyone else's desires or what people thought about your total immersion in self. Although you were far from an island unto yourself, you were unaware of this. The only thing that mattered was getting your needs met. Ah, the good old days.

Then sometime during your first year of life, you began to recognize a mighty presence outside yourself—Mom or Pop.

When you wanted food, food appeared; when you cried out for touch and affection, presto, you got fondled and cuddled; when you squalled in discomfort, suddenly you were soothed. Gradually you learned that it was in your self-interest to keep this magic genie happy so it would stick around and keep on granting your wishes. Things worked pretty smoothly most of the time and life was good.

Slowly your responses to this other caring entity started to matter. You gave up crying when your caretaker scolded you in a harsh voice, quit whining when you got shot a withering glance, stopped dead in your tracks when you were promised a lollipop if you sat quietly. A connection was being forged between approval from this other and your happiness and well-being (although, of course, you didn't consciously make the association). You began to recognize that when your caretakers approved of what you were doing it made them happy, and their happiness made them more inclined to respond to your needs, which made you happy. Conversely, you recognized that when they disapproved of your actions, they grew unhappy and were less inclined to grant your wishes.

See where I'm going with this: All of us learned to be people pleasers to a greater or lesser extent to garner approval in order to survive. Hardwired into every human is the desire to keep on living and to do pretty much whatever it takes to make that happen. This hardwiring is not by chance. If we didn't know how to reap approval as infants and children, our race would have become extinct after its first generation. I'm not saying that trying to get into someone's good graces is always healthy; it's not. I am saying that our predisposition toward seeking approval is so ingrained that most of us don't even realize we're driven by it.

What's wrong with being a super people pleaser?

People pleasing, based on approval seeking, clearly has its place when we're dependent on caretakers for survival. After all, we live solely through their largesse (which is pretty darned scary when you consider some of the parents around). For sure, people pleasing was adaptive back in childhood, when receiving approval or not was literally a matter of life and death. The question is whether it has now become so second nature that you respond by people pleasing when it's not only unnecessary but detrimental to your survival. In fact, many adaptive childhood patterns linger too long, threatening adult health and happiness. People pleasing is one of them.

Behaviors occur along a continuum: We smile or frown, laugh or cry, are active or at rest, rush or dawdle, behave aggressively or passively. An emotionally healthy individual experiences the complete spectrum of emotions (not all at one time, I hope) and can engage in a wide range of survival-enhancing behaviors as appropriate. Not only do we get to choose from one extreme or the other, we also can select from all the nifty options in between. When we're young and dependent on caretakers, doing one type of behavior (any one type), such as people pleasing, may be the sole path to well-being, but when we mature and become independent (or, more accurate, mutually dependent or interdependent), using *only* one strategy becomes maladaptive. Adaptation means being flexible and employing a wide range of behaviors as necessary. So people pleasing as one among many methods of getting by is functional, while doing it to the exclusion of all others is dysfunctional. Get it?

People pleasing based on the need and desire for approval goes right to the heart of being a nice girl. It's the core expectation and wish that sums up how you approach life: If you're nice to people, all will be well. That may even be true a good deal of the time. Most folks *do* react kindly to being treated with consideration and caring. But that's not the point. That *they* enjoy you being nice to them does not mean that it's in *your* best interest. My guess is you've already figured that out and that's why you're reading this book.

▌ **GRAB YOUR THINKING CAP** Do you believe that if you're nice to people, all will be well (or some version of this adage)? How strongly do you believe this and why? ▐

What did my parents do to make me a world-class people pleaser?

Whatever they did, most weren't harming you intentionally and had no idea they were doing anything wrong. They were doing what their parents did to them or trying to do the opposite in reaction to their upbringing. The majority acted in ways they believed were right and would help you grow up to be happy and successful. True, some parents were so stuck in their own orbits that they didn't much care about how you turned out and were only trying to make parenting as easy as possible on themselves. But the bulk of moms and dads don't get up each morning and say to themselves, *Gee, how can I screw up little Susie today? I'd better make a list!*

Nevertheless, here are some of the ways this happens. When exploring early socialization, it always pays to start off with role models. If your mother was a people pleaser, you simply copied what she did and had no idea you were getting yourself into deep doo-doo. Many mothers of nice girls are just the sweetest, dearest, most loving women on the planet. They throw their heart and soul into everything they do—except, of course, taking care of themselves. Often they don't have to say a word about the right way to treat others because their behavior speaks volumes. Other times they harshly discourage "selfish" behavior in their children while strongly encouraging other-oriented behavior. Girls get more of this prodding than do boys, so it's no wonder we think we're the cat's meow when we're good as gold.

How did Mom get across her message of ultraniceness? By denying herself pleasure (time to herself, accepting help, buying or doing nice things for herself, etc.), not confronting Dad, giving in to her children's wishes whether they were appropriate or not, being the family and community caretaker, and never saying an ill word against anyone. She may have dropped what she was doing to tend to family members and run herself ragged or into ill health. She may have talked in a sweet, low voice or tried to be funny and upbeat all the time or bitten her lip when she was mistreated or abused. She even may have kept a smile plastered on her face, though you intuited that she was miserable and hated her life.

Maybe she tried to smooth over family squabbles and begged everyone, "Please, why can't we all get along?" There's a good chance she was overly polite, looked the other way at hurtful behaviors, couldn't tolerate her own negative feelings, and focused on seeing the best in others in order to feel okay. She needed the approval or love of her children or else she felt like a bad parent and her motivation was as much to be loved as to be loving.

Sad to say, not every mother tried to be nice. Some were too consumed with their own problems—depression, mental illness, or substance abuse—and had little leftover energy for kindness and charity. They managed to take care of your physical needs as best they could, but you didn't get much in the way of love and nurturing. Perhaps your mother was moody, controlling, demanding, critical, self-centered, manipulative, or even cruel; being nice obviously was not her strong suit. Maybe Dad was the saint or maybe he was just as bad as Mom (or worse). On the other hand, if he was always trying to get into Mom's good graces by pacifying her and making nice, you might have modeled yourself (consciously or unconsciously) after him rather than her.

▐ **GRAB YOUR THINKING CAP** Have you become a people pleaser to be similar to or different from your parents? ▐

How exactly does my people pleasing shine forth in different situations?

Because you're so used to being other-oriented and focusing on people's (external) approval over self- (internal) approval, you probably have no idea how many ways you try to curry favor. Can you guess how I immediately suspect that a new client is a people pleaser? I pay attention to how many times she says "please," "thank you," and "I'm sorry." I watch her drop her eyes rather than look me in the eye when she makes a request and her lips curl into a smile when she apologizes. I have to tell you that working with nice girls in therapy is a joy and I delight in them because they're so eager to please me and easy to work with. Not only that, I don't have to work hard to figure out what their problem is. It's right there in front of us both. (And, hey, those of you who are in therapy, feel free to ask your therapist if she or he spotted you from the get-go by your niceness.)

But you're not nice only to therapists. Gosh, no—you're nice to *everyone*! Here are some other-oriented questions and scenarios to ponder.

With family

Do you more often than not defer to your spouse or partner? Are you fearful your children won't love you if you punish or say no to them? Do you try to anticipate family members' needs so they don't have to make direct requests? Do you want to jump out of your skin when your kids are arguing and instead automatically leap into the fray to make peace rather than let them settle differences themselves (except when a life is at stake)? Do you suffer extreme agita when there's tension between you and your partner and become preoccupied with making it all better?

Try to admit how much you need to be loved and approved of by your partner and children. It may be difficult to accept your neediness and vulnerability, but at least you'll be responding authentically (perhaps even to please me!). I have never met a nice girl who has equal power in her romantic relationships and have rarely met one who doesn't have difficulty disciplining her children (if she has them) for fear of not being liked by them. If you walk on eggshells around a partner or your kids, tense at their negative reactions, refrain from speaking your mind because they'll go pouty or get riled up, or more often than not deny your needs in order to meet theirs, you're going way, way overboard in the people-pleasing department. There's nothing wrong with your desire to be loved and accepted, but when that becomes *all* that's important and drives most of your behavior, it prohibits you from becoming a complete person (not to mention that it sets a poor example for your children).

Generally the people you want to please most in your family are your parents or your partner and children, and you often take care of them by working hard to fix their problems. They know how antsy you get around messes and how you love to be recognized as Ms. Fix It. What they probably don't realize is how important this role is for you in getting approval. You know what will win you the gold stars and stay stuck in the role, not because you necessarily enjoy it and certainly not because it's good for you, but in order to hear how wonderful and valuable you are and how much everyone loves you for taking such good care of them.

If you don't believe me, try butting out or telling people to stop pestering you with their problems. Try confronting them for making messes and hold them responsible for acting like victims or jerks. See how much approval and love you receive from them then. What I'm saying is that you may not realize that you perform the caretaker role in your family to get approval and keep people happy, that *that* is your underlying motivation. It's fine, of course, if you intervene in some situations, as long as you're picking and choosing your battles and others are doing their fair share. If not, consider that you might have sought out the role because it's how you get a pat on your halo.

▌GRAB YOUR THINKING CAP What do you think will happen if you stop pleasing others and start pleasing yourself? ▐

With friends

What's wrong with pleasing friends? you might ask. They're nice to you, you're nice to them, and everything's kosher. There's absolutely nothing wrong in trying to please friends. In fact, I highly encourage it—as long as it's not a one-sided affair and you're able to be completely genuine with them, that is, as long as it's okay for you *not* to please them as well. For instance, can you tell them you won't be around for Naomi's annual New Year's bash this year because your new beau is taking you to the Ritz? Is it okay not to volunteer to organize Jenna's birthday party since you've done it the last six years? Could you scream or cry for a change instead of cracking jokes and being the comedian who tries to cheer up everyone else? Can you back out of a commitment to go to a movie with enough advance notice because you've been running flat out all week and are dead on your feet? Might some other parent have playdates for the kids at her house for a while because you're recuperating from surgery and need to rest? Could you have forty minutes of airtime and your friend five minutes instead of the other way around like usual?

Are you catching my drift? The idea isn't to stop trying to please friends but to expand your way of relating to them and let them see other sides of you, such as being vulnerable, inadequate, ditzy, unmotivated, grumpy, sad, self-nurturing, or angry. A true friend tries to please you as much as you try to please her. She also lets you be you with all your warts. She doesn't lay unrealistic expectations on you and expect you to be her mother. If you're always trying to please friends, how do you know if they're true blue? You'll know only if you can be yourself and they still like you. If they don't, they're not good friends, simple as that.

▐ **GRAB YOUR THINKING CAP** Are your friendships one-sided in that you do most of the pleasing? What would happen if you stopped working so hard to get acceptance and approval? What would happen if you showed your complete, authentic, flawed self? ▐

With dates

It's natural when we meet people for the first time to put our best foot forward. It's silly to rush out sporting all your worst traits in the hopes that someone will overlook them and love you anyway. In the beginning of relationships, you might let dates pick the restaurant or the movie, try to be flexible about get-togethers, share only appropriate or not too horrifying facts about yourself. What you want to stay alert to is whether your date is making the same effort. Are you being grossly dishonest just to be liked while your date doesn't seem to give a fig what you think of his rudeness or rants? Are you going so overboard to please that your date is taking advantage and quickly getting used to being deferred to? Have you noticed that whenever you don't agree, you're the one who feels pressure to defend yourself or backpedal while your date is fine holding the line?

You may have heard that we learn all we need to about romantic partners early on in the relationship, and I couldn't agree more. If you're dating someone with whom you can let your guard down and there's an equal, easy give-and-take between you, you've at least picked someone who can tolerate and enjoy the real you. However, if you feel an inner pressure that he or she might get angry or reject you if you say the wrong thing, *watch out*! This kind of behavior does not change. So trust your instinct and don't keep trying to please someone who seems indifferent. If they're that way now, he or she will only get worse as the relationship deepens and more is at stake.

■ **GRAB YOUR THINKING CAP** Can you be you with a date, or are you conscious of always trying to please? What happens when you disagree or challenge your partner in a relationship? ■

At work

Just as we don't get to pick our parents, we generally don't get to choose our boss. You get whom you get and have to make the best of it. In an ideal world, you'd have a boss who let you have your say, allowed you to vent your feelings, solicited your opinions, and showered you with praise and compliments. (When you find this boss, let me know. I'd like to work for her!) Most bosses aren't ogres, but they're not out to win a popularity contest either. They're paid to do a job and, if you're lucky, they're tolerable and not mean. A typical boss has likable and unlikable qualities.

That said, there are some real sociopaths and abusers out there who are not to be trifled with. When you sense that your boss is seriously disturbed and get this same feedback from others, not only at work but also outside work, it's time to get out as quickly as you can. Even if you can't leave right away, see if you can be transferred to another department or site or get a different superior. This is important for every employee's mental health, but it's especially vital for people pleasers who often don't recognize sickos and power abusers and could bust a gut trying to make them happy. The problem is you either can't make them happy or doing so robs you of your soul. If you're in this situation, start looking for a way out.

Psychopaths aside, many bosses are simply stressed out, critical people who do an adequate job but have lousy people skills. Some you can work around and some you can't. You may do well with them, as long as you toe the line. But the minute you challenge them and they get angry, you're crushed. You feel betrayed, anxious, and helpless and don't know what to do with your feelings. Sometimes it may even make you literally sleepless and sick. Non–people pleasers objectively consider their situation and strategize about what to do and say. But people pleasers get so twitchy about loss of approval and acceptance that they're almost paralyzed emotionally. If you're in this kind of situation, you need outside, objective help not only to get over your need for approval but also to figure out what to do.

The same situations crop up with colleagues and subordinates. You meet some colleagues and feel as if you've known them your whole life. Others aren't easy to get to know and keep to themselves. People pleasers need to be careful in these circumstances not to mistake aloofness and a need for privacy for rejection. You haven't necessarily done something wrong because someone isn't interested in cozying up to you or doesn't notice or seem to care much about you. Consider that it may be his or her problem and that you don't have to spend the rest of your days questing after acceptance.

▌ GRAB YOUR THINKING CAP Are you a people pleaser with your boss, colleagues, superiors, subordinates, clients? Are you in a situation in which your boss is verbally abusive and you need to get out? What are you waiting for? ▌

In the community

I'm fortunate in my life to have met amazing women (and men) who would stand out in any community. They're the movers and shakers, the ones who are out there writing letters to the editor, picketing and demonstrating, ministering to the poor and unfortunate, advocating for the powerless, and putting their ethical and political beliefs into action and on the line. Some activists are working for the good of the community and truly are motivated to create a better world for themselves, their children, and future generations. These people are driven by altruistic inner forces and basically don't care a plug nickel if you approve of what they're doing or not.

Then there are people pleasers who are out there because they believe it's their duty or are seeking approval for it. Maybe Mom drilled into you that you *must* help the downtrodden to be a good citizen or Dad insisted you give your allowance to the needy. If the way these demands were made included a parent severely disapproving of (or even punishing) you or showing excessive disappointment in you for not living up to unrealistic standards, you could, as an adult, still be seeking the approval of parents who are long dead and buried (or at least hold no power over you). Let's face it, getting involved in your neighborhood, community, or world is a positive activity and I'm not trying to discourage you from doing so—it feels good to give of ourselves. However, if you tend toward people pleasing, it's important to examine your motives and make sure you're doing good work because of how it makes you feel and not so the world will love you more.

▌ **GRAB YOUR THINKING CAP** If you work in your community as a volunteer or activist, what is your honest motivation? Do you expect people to admire and approve of you, or are you doing it because you believe it's the right thing to do? ▌

How does being a people pleaser drive me to be queen of the carbohydrates?

Emotionally healthy individuals feel good in the moment and flattered when folks compliment and praise them. They don't need the approval of their partner, friends, children, family, neighbors, or boss to do the right thing and engage in activities they enjoy. If they get it, all well and good; if not, so what. Healthy people might get upset when they don't feel valued or appreciated, but they can go a long way toward validating themselves when others don't do it for them, and external validation is icing on their cake. If they're regularly undervalued, they speak up to find out why and let others know that they'd like to be appreciated a bit more.

However, when you've built your whole life around seeking approval and acceptance, it's devastating when you don't get it. It can send you into a downward spiral or a tailspin that's difficult to recover from. It can generate anxiety and depression and even make you feel suicidal. Sometimes when you've worked hard to curry favor and don't receive it, you feel profoundly disappointed, worthless, empty, betrayed, and as if there's no point in living. This is the problem with seeking external reward exclusively: If you don't get it, you feel completely done in. You may even feel resentful and enraged and not understand where this surge of intense feeling comes from.

And what do you do to avoid or lessen these feelings? You eat, of course. You think, *Well, if no one's going to reward me, I'll just reward myself with a treat.* If you can't fill up on compliments, you fill yourself up on calories. People can disappoint you, but food never does, so what the heck. You tell yourself, *I deserve something good to eat,* which is of course the truth but not a great way to decide whether to have pizza or not. Sure, you deserve to be loved and lauded, but that has nothing to do with food. When you really believe that you're deserving, food doesn't enter into the equation because your reward is your own good feelings about yourself.

Food fills the void left by lack of approval, but only temporarily. When you're done eating, you're still left with empty feelings of inadequacy and insecurity, made worse by mistrust in yourself for eating when you weren't hungry or overeating when you were. You're still yearning for external reinforcement and have compounded the problem by not focusing on what you can actively do to make yourself feel better—reminding yourself of your worth, realizing that your judgment of yourself is more important than how others judge you, and accepting that seeking approval outside the self is generally a fruitless endeavor.

▌ **GRAB YOUR THINKING CAP** What do you do when you've failed to receive the acceptance, love, or approval you seek? How do you abuse food in these situations? What is it you're seeking through eating? ▌

I've been privileged to see many nice girls turn around people-pleasing behavior in a short time. It's not easy, but it's not as hard as you might think. It takes reflection, awareness, insight, and what's called an observant ego, that is, the ability to act and assess your actions simultaneously. Using your observing ego on a date might involve noticing how you're fawning or keeping your opinions to yourself because you sense your companion hates to be challenged. Or recognizing that you didn't send your son to his room because you can't stand how angry he gets at you when you punish him. Or realizing that you couldn't refuse to give your drug-addict brother a handout because he so looks to his big sis as a savior. People pleasing is as addictive as any other behavior that lights up your brain's reward center, but change becomes easier when you focus on approving of yourself. Work on lighting up your own pleasure center!

NO MORE NICE GIRL MANIFESTO FOR PEOPLE PLEASING

DO

- Share your authentic feelings with people you feel safe with.

- Cultivate family and friend relationships with folks who can accept you as you are and to whom you can speak honestly and directly.

- Try to understand where your people-pleasing behavior comes from in your childhood.

- Analyze your work situation and see if you are setting yourself up for excessive approval seeking and confrontation avoidance.

- Allow your children to be angry with you so that they can learn that it's okay to be angry and continue to be loved.

- Explain to your partner why you fear being honest (unless your partner will retaliate and hurt you, in which case either seek counseling or get out of the relationship).

- Expect friends to love you in spite of your flaws.

- Make sure that your community work is being done not because you feel you should do it or will be rewarded for it, but because it feels pretty neat in your heart.

- Stop expecting acceptance, approval, praise, or love from others for what you do and instead give it to yourself.

- Stop saying nice things so folks will like you or won't be angry with you.

- Expect that you'll hurt people's feelings and they'll get over it.

- Practice saying no more often and think long and hard before saying yes.

DON'T

- Worry if someone you meet doesn't like you.

- Expect praise and compliments for everything you do as if you are a child who needs constant encouragement.

- Smile when you don't feel like it just to cheer up someone.

- Say yes when the more self-nurturing answer is no.

- Stay in an abusive home, social, or work situation in which you're walking on eggshells around a person who is critical, abusive, or in other ways habitually hurtful.

- Overdo just to make other people happy when it doesn't seem right for you.

- Keep silent and make excuses for people who regularly behave badly.

- Let hurt fester because you're afraid of sharing negative feelings.

- Catastrophize about folks not getting over hurt feelings, which are part of life.

- Say "please," "thank you," and "I'm sorry" unless it's appropriate.

To do today

The next time you do something you're proud of, don't ask anyone what they think, but focus on what you think of your behavior.

Meet One of the Nice Girls

Maura now

Maura, recently turned twenty-two, came to see me because she didn't want to end up like her four brothers and sisters whom she describes as "pitiful wrecks" who have a slew of mental health and substance abuse problems. She says that even in her worst depressive state she's the healthiest member of her family, which makes her feel grim and hopeless.

Artistically gifted, she's just received a BA in fine arts and is one talented lady from what I've seen of her art in photographs of her paintings. To support herself while she paints amazing murals (mostly of women who are full of intense emotion), she's cobbled together a bunch of jobs—dog sitter and walker, house cleaner, and photographer's assistant—which give her control over her life and time to paint when she feels like it.

An avid self-help reader, she's on an antidepressant, which lessens her dark moods but doesn't prevent her from eating and drinking to help modulate them. She readily admits she has both eating and drinking problems but can't imagine life without using "something to breathe some life into me." She's tried to stop drinking, but the longest she's been alcohol free is three months. However, she has cut down quite a bit since graduation, believing she has to be more responsible with "my crazy work schedule." She yo-yos between dieting and binge eating, has four sizes of clothing in her closet, and wants off the food merry-go-round.

I spotted Maura as a nice girl the minute she walked in the door—fifteen minutes late. She'd called from her cell phone right before the appointment, breathless and apologizing repeatedly because she'd had a problem with one of her client's dogs. In fact, I could hear her apologizing to the dog owner in the background that she had to leave for an appointment. Then she spent the first five minutes of our session showering me with more "sorry's" and thanked me for seeing her though she was late. Naturally, she ended the session swearing to be on time in the future. Guilt and gratitude simply oozed from every pore.

Ironically, when I commented on what a nice girl she seemed to be, she looked positively shocked. "Me, nice?" she exclaimed, "Wow, you're kidding, right?"

Maura as a child

Both Maura's parents are drinkers, and all her older siblings have either substance abuse or mental health problems or both. Her father was a functional alcoholic who often stopped off at a bar after work (as a machinist) until her mother started to join him for cocktail hour to keep him home. Maura swears her mother wouldn't have become an alcoholic if it weren't for her wanting to keep tabs on Dad, a well-known ladies' man who continued to have affairs throughout the marriage. When her parents were sober, they got along fairly well, but all their misgivings and regrets were unleashed when they'd had a few, and Maura and her siblings used to either leave the house or barricade themselves in their bedrooms as soon as the tirades began.

Maura's two older sisters couldn't wait to get out of the house and married early, then continued to remarry unhappily and divorce. One of her brothers is a heroin addict who still lives with their parents and the other has bipolar disorder and multiple addictions and lives in a supervised group home. Maura describes her siblings growing up as "in their own worlds." When she was younger, her sisters hung out with each other, as did her brothers, leaving her alone much of the time. She started drinking and smoking pot when she was twelve and, while her folks were trying to find oblivion downstairs, she was trying to find it in her room. Actually, she's grateful that her parents mostly left her alone because that left her time to draw and paint and "put my pain to paper."

De-nicing Maura

One of my ongoing maneuvers is to call Maura on her apologies when none is necessary or when she overdoes it with "thank you" and "please." This helps her realize how these words pepper her speech and usually leads to talking about how grateful she is when anyone is nice to her. When she speaks of this gratitude, she almost always cries, which generates discussion of how defective she feels and her need to constantly make up for it by being nice to people. The issue of defectiveness is huge for nice girls and we always come back to it as being at the core of her problems.

After much discussion and convincing, Maura begins to attend AA and finds, to her surprise, that she likes it and feels comfortable with the people she meets there. She can't believe they're so much like her. Through AA she starts dating a man who has been sober three years and seems to have his act pretty much together. Maura is happier but doesn't feel worthy of this man and pulls away until he gives up and breaks off the relationship.

This pattern happens repeatedly in therapy and is rooted in her feeling defective and her subsequent low self-esteem. This same pattern dogs her relationship with food and drink. She'll eat normally or healthily for a while, then binge all out for a week and start her diet on a Monday morning. She'll remain sober for months, then go on a bender. We discuss her genetic predisposition to chemicals and why she self-sabotages when she feels good. She's gaining insight slowly, and knows it may take years for her to stop abusing food and alcohol and get her life in order.

What's Next? *In Chapter 10, "Learning to Be Selfish," you'll learn*

- How you came to believe that selfishness is wrong

- How to change your beliefs to be comfortable with selfishness

- Why you never have to worry about turning into a totally selfish person

TEN

Me, Me, Me, Me, Me . . . *Just Practicing!*

Learning to Be Selfish

S o, are you selfish yet? Have you thrown off your nice girl mantle and begun swathing yourself in diamonds and furs? Doubtful. Change takes a long time, an excruciatingly long time. Still, after reading this far, I expect your thinking is starting to shift about just how unselfish you can afford to be, and your nice, soft edges are beginning to sharpen a bit. Good. I expect you may have picked up various ideas from different chapters but that your approach to de-nicing yourself is rather haphazard. Now that you've got your running shoes on, you need a map of how to get where you want to go.

Because change is so scary and overwhelming, I encourage people to take it very slowly and experiment rather than to devise and execute a full-court press to revamp their personality. Nine out of ten times, this makeover-in-a-month burns people out, promotes a success-or-failure model (exactly the type of all-or-nothing thinking you want to get away from), and mobilizes your fears of change all at once. Instead, I favor offering a taste of what's possible and making suggestions. It's not up to me to tell you what to do and how to do it (following instructions *too* well is why you're reading this book in the first place), but for you to find your own route out of Niceville.

That said, there are certain tasks that need to be done before you leave your sugar-coated chains behind. Don't panic—you have the rest of your life to keep inching along, so relax and take the long view. Every baby step that leads you away from perfectionism, people pleasing, silencing yourself, and putting yourself last will decrease your stress level, make you happier, and cut the cord between you and food. Think of it this way: When a baby runs, what happens? She generally picks up so much speed that she falls down, boom, on her tiny fanny. But when she takes small, cautious steps, she eventually gets where she wants to go. You are that baby as you grow into a better version of the old you, so tie those pink laces and start walking.

The first thing you have to do is not, as you might assume, focus on your behavior. Remember that earlier I distinguished among beliefs, feelings, and behaviors. Behavior is often the last aspect of self to shift; what comes first is beliefs. The cognitive-behavioral model says that beliefs produce feelings and behavior and that recasting beliefs transforms how you feel and what you do. So although you'll be working on three fronts at once, most of your initial efforts will be on developing a sound, rational belief system that will, in turn, promote healthy feelings and behaviors that are appropriate and effective.

For now, let's return to the beliefs, emotions, and behaviors of nice girls.

WHAT YOU BELIEVE

- I am responsible for people's happiness.

- I need to be upbeat and cheerful, and make people feel better.

- People will fall apart without my help.

- If I say what I feel, people will be hurt and won't like me.

- If I stop being overly nice, people won't accept me.

- I have to be perfect, including how I look and act and what I say.

- I need praise from others to feel okay about myself.

- Saying no to others' requests means I'm selfish.

- Putting myself first means I'm self-centered and don't care about others.

- I'm not a good person unless I'm being helpful or productive.

WHAT YOU FEEL

- I can't bear when people are in distress.

- I feel guilty letting people down by disappointing them or not meeting their needs.

- I feel driven to keep people's spirits up and to prevent them from suffering.

- I can't stand hurting other people's feelings.

- I'm scared people won't like me if I stop being overly nice.

- I'm determined to be/look/act perfect because I hate failing or making mistakes.

- I feel inadequate and insecure unless people shower me with praise and compliments, although I mostly don't believe them.

- I hate the thought that I might be selfish and feel awful about myself when I think I am.

- I feel guilty if I take care of myself rather than other people.

- I feel lost and useless unless I'm doing for others or being useful.

HOW YOU BEHAVE

- I listen endlessly to people's problems, offer solutions, and give advice.

- I do favors for people even when I don't have the time or the energy and they don't reciprocate.

- I'm a smiley face and cover my negative feelings to appear upbeat.

- I say things I don't mean and do things I don't want to do simply to avoid hurting someone's feelings.

- I avoid confronting and challenging people and am a yes-girl.

- I obsess about looking/acting/saying things perfectly and would rather die than make a mistake.

- I rarely stand up for myself, set and stick to clear and firm boundaries, or put myself first.

- Because I don't know when enough is enough, I overdo even when it stresses me to the max.

- Guilt drives most of my behavior and it's so automatic I don't even realize it.

- I don't know how to stop being so darned nice to people.

❚ **GRAB YOUR THINKING CAP** Is this still what you believe, feel, and do, or have you already made some changes? What are they and in which of the three categories do they fall? ❚

Assuming that you haven't made a total transformation, let's examine your beliefs and see where you're on the right track and where you're stuck in a rut. Although the beliefs listed above are not all-inclusive—I invite you to spend time creating ones that are unique to you—they do cover most of the ways that nice girls get caught up in stinkin' thinkin'. The goal is to recognize your beliefs as irrational and reframe them (that is, turn them) into rational beliefs that will promote healthy emotions and actions. *Capisce?* Good. Let's examine these beliefs one by one and make them rational.

I am responsible for people's happiness

Really? Is that everyone in the entire world, or just the people you know? Does it include me, too? If so, how soon can you drop by? And when you say "responsible," does that mean for everything a person ever is and does or for only some things? Ladies, can you see where I'm going here? I don't know about you, but it's all I can handle being responsible for myself and, occasionally, my cat. Everyone else is on her own.

If you truly believe that other people's happiness is your responsibility, then you, like Superwoman, face a never-ending battle to defeat the forces of evil. Of course, it's nonsense that you're responsible for anyone's happiness or welfare except children, animals, or folks who are incapable of rational judgment due to cognitive impairment or medical or mental conditions that inhibit their ability to make sound decisions for themselves. People who *can* think clearly but *choose* not to are a different story. Occasionally, you may decide to help them out, especially if they're working very hard to take better care of themselves and have veered off track, but even then you're still not responsible for them. They are responsible for them.

So here are rational reframings for *I am responsible for people's happiness*:

- I am responsible for my own happiness.

- Each person is responsible for his or her own happiness.

- What people choose to say or do is not my responsibility.

- Being responsible for other people's happiness doesn't allow them to be responsible for themselves.

I need to be upbeat and cheerful, and make people feel better

Who says? Did I miss that lesson in my fourth-grade citizenship class? First of all, you don't *need* to be any which way. The only thing you absolutely have to do in life is die. Sometimes you will naturally feel upbeat and cheerful. Other times you will equally naturally feel crabby, cranky, glum, gloomy, and pissy. Such is life. Think yin and yang, up and down, complementarity, and balance. If there's anything you *need*, it's to allow yourself a full range of emotions. Some people are inherently cheerful, mostly due to their DNA and sometimes in spite of having a wretched childhood. Then there are other people who appear to have lived a reasonably decent life but are perpetual pessimists.

Anyway, why must you change your emotions and how you behave in order for someone else to feel better? You might want to give yourself a little talking to when your bad mood hangs on for days and days and shake yourself out of it, but that's enough work for one person. Each of us has to lift our own spirits and, if we can't, well, that's the way the cookie crumbles. Moreover, why *must* people feel better? There are many times when it's normal and healthy to feel bad—after an intimate dies, when you have a grave illness, when disaster has befallen you or your family, about the state of the world. Perhaps the problem isn't really about someone else feeling bad but how that makes you feel: helpless, uncomfortable, antsy to fix the problem.

Try on these rational beliefs instead of *I need to be upbeat and cheerful, and make people feel better*:

- I don't need to feel any certain way.

- How I feel is based not on my reactions to others but on my internal cues.

- Other people are responsible for making themselves feel better.

- Sometimes feeling bad is normal and healthy and what people must experience in the course of life.

People will fall apart without my help

When you say fall apart, what does that look like? Will they take to their beds, need to be hospitalized, have a screaming fit, become ill and die? You may or may not have a clear picture in your head of what "falling apart" looks like. More often than not, what you have is a vague feeling that things will not go well for someone. What you're usually afraid of is that if this person "falls apart," you'll suffer somehow—bear the brunt of her ill will, feel pressured to take better care of him, receive less attention or love from her, or get blamed for his failings.

The second part of this belief implies that you are the only one who can keep Humpty Dumpty together. Is that really true? If so, might that be because you've become a human glue stick with your family / friends / workplace / community? I hate to be the one to break it to you, but in many instances when you think you're indispensable, you're not. If you die tomorrow, someone will probably step in to take your place as Glue Woman, making sure that whoever gets taken care of.

The following rational beliefs make much more sense than *People will fall apart without my help*:

- Other people will step in, if necessary, to help those I can't.

- People will do fine without my help and not fall apart and even find strengths they don't know they have.

- People who fall apart usually can be put back together.

- Even if someone falls apart, that doesn't mean I'm going to suffer.

If I say what I feel, people will be hurt and won't like me
Okay, let's play this one out. So you say what's on your mind and someone is offended. Why does that automatically mean he won't like you? Maybe he'll feel neutral or be ever grateful that you shared honestly with him. Or perhaps he will be put off or insulted, but he'll get over it. Worst case is that he won't like you. Then what? He'll attack you with a machete or pitch you into a river? If you're in a nonabusive (emotional, sexual, or physical) relationship, you're likely to remain safe even if someone decides he hates you momentarily. Yes, some people will retaliate or pull away from you, but they're in the minority—and you're slowly going to work yourself away from them and avoid people like them, aren't you?

The key here is your fear of what your life will be like if someone doesn't like you. You've catastrophized and blown the concept way out of proportion. Other than when you're highly dependent on someone (as in childhood), it really doesn't matter much if people like you: the clerk at the checkout counter, your neighbor's sister's boyfriend, the principal at your child's school, your husband's golf partner, Uncle Fred who flies in once a year for Christmas dinner, your therapist's secretary, your mechanic. You need to answer this question:

How will so-and-so not liking me substantially affect my life? Even if your parents or children don't like you, you'll survive, and if you're partner doesn't, well, there's more than one fish in the sea.

Give these rational beliefs a whirl instead of *If I say what I feel, people will be hurt and won't like me*:

- If I say what I feel, people may or may not be hurt.

- If I say what I feel, people may or may not like me.

- I will survive hurting people's feelings and they'll survive, too.

- I will survive people not liking me when I say what I feel.

If I stop being overly nice, people won't accept me

This belief is similar to your fear of not being liked. The first thing to consider is why being accepted is so important that you'd develop a whole dysfunctional way of interacting with people around it. Are you afraid of being excluded, cast aside, left out? What will happen then? Will something terrible befall you because you're alone or on the outside looking in? Most of us would prefer to be accepted by most people, but that's not possible. After all, you can't possibly be valued equally by someone from the Ku Klux Klan and the NAACP. As an adult, you get to decide whose acceptance is important to you and, to repeat, that cannot be everyone.

The wish to be accepted often comes from wanting to be loved, valued, and included as is. You may not feel accepting of others who aren't nice and you may not value yourself when you're not nice, but others might not care very much and love you anyway. Think about that, and be careful not to confuse how you feel about others or yourself with how they might feel about you (in psychology, by the way, this process is called projection).

There are a number of ways to reframe *If I stop being overly nice, people won't accept me* that make a whole lot more sense:

• If I stop being overly nice, some people will accept me and some won't and that's okay.

• I can tolerate not being accepted.

• Everyone need not accept me for me to live a happy, fulfilling life.

• It's important for me to accept me when I'm not nice because I'm being genuine.

I have to be perfect, including how I look and act and what I say

You already know a lot about the dangers of perfectionism, so here's your chance to road-test your beliefs. One force behind wanting to be perfect is control, as in, *if I look/act/appear perfect, nothing bad will befall me*. It's time to question whether this is true. Has striving toward ideals really warded off bad things from happening to you? Doubtful. Awful things happen to everyone, whether we're good or bad, doing our best or worst, a stellar human being, a shark, or a mess.

The "have to" you feel is the need to control your life. We do have command over some parts of living. We should definitely make thoughtful choices and consider consequences whenever possible. But even then we can't prevent life from bringing us raging storms when we're hoping for sunny skies. Rather than believe you need to be perfect, focus on experiencing your feelings, thinking clearly, using good judgment, and surrounding yourself with emotionally healthy people. The key is to focus on what you can do now for a positive outcome. Your life will turn out better and you won't need to yearn so much for perfection. Believe you can handle anything that comes along, and you'll *always* be prepared.

Some positive reframings of *I have to be perfect, including how I look and act and what I say* are:

- I don't have to be perfect—ever—and can look, act, and say what I want.

- There's no such thing as human perfection.

- I need to build internal resources and external support to feel okay in bad times, rather than strive for perfection to ward them off.

- It's healthier to like and accept my flawed self than to try to be perfect.

I need praise from others to feel okay about myself

Wherever you got this notion, you should return it and get your money back. The point to examine here is what you think will happen if you don't feel okay about yourself: Will you feel inadequate, insecure, unloved, depressed, suicidal? By depending on others to "make" you feel good about yourself, you've missed opportunities to build up your own reserve of good feelings or strengthen your ability to feel okay about yourself by yourself. By insisting that you need praise from others, you undermine your confidence in your ability to be emotionally resourceful, exactly what will get you over life's rough patches.

When you believe you need praise, you're bound to keep pursuing it. But it's never really enough to fill you up (that can be done only by you) and, moreover, it makes you keep coming back for more. Pretty soon you feel like a mouse on a wheel that goes round and round. The only way to get off is to tend to your own bad feelings, look inward to lift your spirits, and keep doing things to make yourself proud of you. Looking to others automatically undermines an authentic and lasting sense of basic okayness.

Rather than believe *I need praise from others to feel okay about myself*, try these rational beliefs on for size:

- I can feel okay without praise from others.

- I can give myself praise to feel better.

- Nothing feels as good as self-approval.

- Feeling okay about myself happens only when I have self-trust and confidence in my own abilities.

Saying no to others' requests means I'm selfish

Somewhere along the way two things that do not go together—saying no and being selfish—got hooked together in your world and you haven't been able to unhook them. Saying no to other people *all the time* means you care about yourself over others. Saying no sometimes or occasionally means you're healthy, normal, and in balance! No one can possibly say yes to everything people ask of them and remain sane. Think of it this way: Saying no to others is really about saying yes to yourself.

There are people who make reasonable requests and people whose demands are so ludicrous they should be laughed at.

Many people have no idea how impossible they are; others know and couldn't care less. Like children, they want what they want when they want it. Well, tough noogies. Listen up: Most people who accuse you of being selfish are either trying to deflect the fact that they're the selfish ones, or are terrified of the concept of putting themselves first and feel threatened by your having a stronger sense of self.

The first thing to do in considering requests is to ask yourself whether they are rational, fair, and doable. The second is to reflect on how saying yes will *realistically* affect you, them, and the relationship. The third is to think about how saying no will manifest into consequences. If you're not taking into account all these factors, you're bound to overdo.

Excellent rational reframings of *Saying no to others' requests means I'm selfish* include:

- Saying no to others doesn't mean I'm selfish because only I can decide if I am.

- Saying no to others means I'm saying yes to myself.

- I can't possibly meet everyone's requests and take care of myself.

- I am not selfish if I refuse unreasonable, unfair requests.

Putting myself first means I'm self-centered and don't care about others

More confusion on your part. You aren't self-centered because you put yourself first. I'll say it again: You're healthy. Selfishness is on a continuum from self-centered to other-centered. Neither extreme is the right place to be all the time. The idea is to be fluidly in balance so that you can comfortably do for self *and* others. People who are terrified of being thought self-centered (or thinking of themselves that way) go too far to the other extreme.

Caring about other people can be shown in many ways, not just putting them first. Often you have to use tough love and take a hard tack *because* you can see what's best for someone even if she can't see it herself. Naturally, this situation occurs a lot with parenting children or taking care of elderly parents who have lost some cognitive ability. These are difficult circumstances where you might feel crummy doing something you know hurts them but is best for you, like putting an impaired parent in a nursing home near you or moving your kids because you landed a terrific job in another state.

These rational beliefs are a good replacement for *Putting myself first means I'm self-centered and don't care about others*:

- Putting myself first means I care about myself.

- Only I can decide if I'm self-centered.

- I can put myself first and also care about other people.

- I would be self-centered if I always put myself first, but I don't.

I'm not a good person unless I'm being helpful or productive

What is a good person, anyway? What I think is a good person is not necessarily what you or another reader might think. We each have to be acceptable to ourselves in our own eyes. Good might mean someone who is present, enjoys life to the fullest, is creative and full of joy. It also might mean helpful or productive. But no one is one way all the time. Being helpful and productive are wonderful traits, but being that way 24/7 doesn't give you a chance to recharge your batteries and take care of yourself.

This belief smacks of socialization that encouraged always giving and never taking or constantly being on the go without resting, of putting out rather than taking in. People who are always endeavoring to be helpful or productive are way off track. Their ideals are too high—and probably so is their stress level. The goal is to balance being helpful to others *and* self, to spend time productively and goofing off, to work and play. Too often the only way you achieve downtime is through abusing food. Stop being so helpful and productive and find ways to nourish yourself with real fun, pleasure, and contentment.

Time to change *I'm not a good person unless I'm being helpful or productive* to the following:

- I'm a good person whether or not I'm helpful or productive.

- Being helpful or productive doesn't make me good or bad.

- I can be a good person when I'm doing nothing and helping no one.

- I need to balance giving to others and giving to myself.

❚ **GRAB YOUR THINKING CAP** Which beliefs ring truest for you? Which ones do you expect will be hardest to change? ❚

The work of reframing beliefs is crucial to changing your nice girl behavior. You'll soon see that reframed, rational beliefs promote feeling less guilty, inadequate, insecure, frightened, resentful, and undervalued. They form the foundation for a healthier self. As your feelings shift, so will your behavior. If you don't believe it's selfish to make space and time for yourself, you won't feel guilty when you do and will take better care of yourself. If you're sure it's okay to hurt people's feelings in the service of taking care of your own, you won't feel so scared to speak up and will have a more mature, healthy relationship with others. If you don't believe you have to prevent other people from falling apart, you'll feel more relaxed, and reduced stress will lead to decreased unwanted eating. If you're certain you can function without being perfect, you'll feel less internal pressure and have more time to have fun and enjoy life.

But is it really okay to be selfish?

You're going to have to decide for yourself. Maybe it'll help to examine where you developed your terror of the *s* word. Of course, in order to do that, we're going to have to travel back in time and see what you learned about selfishness growing up. There's probably not a family on earth in which a parent, at some time, doesn't accuse a child of being selfish, because, well, children are! They're naturally focused on their own needs. We *do* have to be taught to care about and share with others, to take their feelings into account, to balance their needs with ours. Although we're assuredly hardwired with the potential ability to live cooperatively and interdependently, it generally doesn't happen on its own. And that's where effective parenting makes all the difference.

If your parents reprimanded you only when you were really being selfish—like when you wouldn't let your friends play with *any* of your stuffed animals or *never* let your sister borrow your bike—you learned that thinking only of yourself brought parental disapproval. Moreover, if your parents modeled being appropriately kind, caring, and giving and praised you when you acted in these ways, you received positive reinforcement. If they also told your sister not to hog your bike and your friends to play carefully with your stuffed animals, you learned that there is a natural give-and-take to life and that everyone gets along better when no one is selfish.

However, if you were accused of being selfish when you wanted to do something and your parents didn't want you to—say, you wanted to go out and play and they wanted you to vacuum the house because they didn't feel like it—you picked up the message that having your own needs is selfish. Dysfunctional families excel at giving the wrong message about many things, and among them is who has what needs. Healthy families are child-centered not parent-centered, to a point. In unhealthy families, parents regularly put their needs before their children's.

Most likely you were called selfish but rarely were. Often parents who regularly blame their children (and each other) for being selfish are themselves narcissists. To avoid seeing this trait in themselves, they instead shift the blame onto you. The truth is that very self-involved parents sometimes produce children who are totally other-oriented because they're scared of being accused of selfishness. Or kids go out of their way to become selfless and altruistic because they can't stand the thought of being like their narcissistic parents.

Narcissism is a personality trait in which people have so little sense of self and rightness of being that they go in the other direction and come off as boastful and grandiose. Narcissists easily get emotionally injured and insulted, must always be right, tend to blame and be highly critical of others, and let themselves off the hook when they should take responsibility. They put so much energy into warding off threats to self from others and feeling okay about themselves that they have little left over for anyone else. Put another way, they are so busy taking care of self that there's no room for anybody else unless it boosts their feelings about themselves.

Narcissistic parents often produce nice girls (and boys). If you had two narcissistic parents, you had a double whammy of authentic selfishness and all its accompanying destructive attitudes and behaviors. This is hard stuff to shake off, especially if your parents are still living and you have to deal with them in all their self-absorbed, entitled glory. The goal is not to blame them for how they brought you up (they did the best they could, although it wasn't good enough), but for you to understand the misguided beginnings of your concept of selfishness.

One other point. Very often a flagrantly narcissistic parent is also a nonstop do-gooder: She makes dinners for the neighbors who lost their house in a fire, takes in stray animals, rises to power in the community as a volunteer, spends hours in charity work. However, along with these good works (and, make no mistake, these are good works) comes a need to brag about them. These are not self-effacing, humble people who never mention that they were Parent of the Year or donated $25,000 to put an addition on their son's school. They're the people who want (and make sure they get) the credit. So, sadly, their good works are often tarnished by bragging and a need for recognition, which is off-putting. Children sense this and often vow to be unlike them, so that they paradoxically end up holding on to the charitable nature of their parents while eschewing their credit seeking. Instead, they try to be humble and self-effacing.

People who are *self-centered* and *self-absorbed*, generally a function of narcissism, talk a lot about themselves and redirect conversation back to *their* problems and *their* accomplishments. You know the old joke: *Well, enough about me. What do you think of me?* Of course, they don't see their self-absorption and would vehemently deny it if the whole world got together and voted them Narcissist of the Year. So the good news is that if you *think* you're self-centered and selfish, you probably aren't!

NO MORE NICE GIRL MANIFESTO FOR SELFISHNESS

DO

- Act in ways that exude self-care and high self-esteem.

- Try being naughty and see what happens.

- Break the habit of taking care of other people at your own expense.

- Make sure you have totally rational beliefs about selfishness.

- Notice people who are truly selfish and the difference between you and them.

- Recognize that you can become more selfish and still be a giving, caring person.

- Stop looking for other people to praise you and start validating yourself.

- Define for yourself what makes you a good person rather than seek other folks' opinions.

- Take responsibility for your happiness and let other people be responsible for their own.

- Allow your moods and emotions to emerge naturally and don't try to shape them into cheerful and upbeat when they're not.

- Focus more on accepting yourself rather than gaining acceptance from others.

- Experiment with saying no.

- Allow yourself to hurt people's feelings if it happens in the process of taking care of your own.

- Challenge or ignore people who call you selfish.

DON'T

- Try to be all things to all people just to avoid the label of selfish.

- Accept other people's definition of what makes you good, kind, and unselfish.

- Avoid downtime because you feel pressure to be productive and useful.

- Believe that the only way you can show caring for people is by fixing their problems or helping them out.

- Hang around with truly selfish, narcissistic people.

- Ignore self-care because taking care of yourself makes you feel selfish.

- Equate selfish with effective self-care.

- Worry so much about what people think of you.

- Let others blame you for their problems.

- Be concerned with turning into a totally selfish person, because it'll never happen.

Now that you have the dos and don'ts of selfishness straight, it's time to put all you've learned together. Take a few deep breaths and don't worry if you haven't figured out all you need to do to de-nice yourself. You didn't become nice overnight and you're not going to shift into balance without plenty of hard work, patience, compassion, humor, self-reflection, and discomfort. And, remember, you don't have to give up being nice just to stop being a nice girl!

To do today

Do something selfish—say no to an unreasonable demand, take time for yourself even though someone else needs you, or make yourself happy even though it makes someone else unhappy.

Meet One of the Nice Girls

Miriam now

Miriam is a fifty-eight-year-old ball of fire who comes from a line of firebrands. She is gay, which is not an issue for her. She entered therapy because she was having difficulty sleeping and was almost too exhausted to continue her host of volunteer activities, which include being an active member of Planned Parenthood and sitting on the board of two nonprofit community agencies. Trained as a lawyer, she provides additional pro bono counseling to just about anyone who needs it—individuals or organizations. In fact, when she interviewed me to see if we would be a good therapeutic match, one of the questions she asked was what volunteer activities I did. Good thing I had a couple to share with her!

Her legal talents are put to good use working for the Service Employees International Union, for which she is one of their main negotiators. She's passionate about her work and values each day by how much she's done for others. Not surprising, she can't understand why everyone doesn't do as much as she does, why they at least don't give back to their community in some small way. When she talks about her job, she never seems tired or put upon and it truly appears to energize her.

As I've told her, however, she lives her life playing only one, long note. She has friends, but when she's with them, they generally talk politics or lament the sorry state of the world. A few times she's come close to what she calls "giving up my independence," but she's always been the one to end the relationship. She doesn't appear lonely, but there is *something* she craves that she lacks, which comes out in her insatiable appetite. Miriam can sit down and polish off huge quantities of food at a time, generally of the carbo variety, and identifies herself as an "Olympian binge eater." When she was younger, she kept weight off by all her running around and playing volleyball, but over the last decade, it's crept up by a few pounds every year. She claims she has no time to exercise, although there's a gym right next to her office.

When I raise the issue of her difficulty sleeping, she becomes agitated that she has a problem she can't fix by applying energy and intelligence. She refuses to take any kind of sleep aid but has recently agreed to try a few herbal remedies. Reluctantly, she admits that the sleeplessness started around the time she realized she was approaching sixty. She said she didn't feel old but feared she couldn't accomplish all she wanted to in her remaining time on earth.

Miriam as a child

She was raised by parents who considered themselves Socialists, and righting society's wrongs was the family mission. During her childhood, both parents had full-time blue collar jobs and still found time to volunteer in the community. In fact, much of the volunteering was done as a family in a local soup kitchen. Her mother loved to bake and gave out freebies to everyone in the neighborhood. Her father, a gifted mediator, settled community disputes.

Miriam knows no other way of living because she rarely saw anything different growing up. Her siblings are all activists or advocates. Most of her parents' friends and extended family shared their values. She was raised on the principle of sharing and giving, that the haves must advocate for and take care of the have-nots, and that we are all our sisters' keepers. Her parents are still thriving in an independent living facility where they sit on the resident council.

De-nicing Miriam

Miriam has so many strengths that they're hard to count, including a deep curiosity about why things are as they are. She's intrigued that her sleeplessness and binge eating might be trying to tell her something about herself, and that becomes the springboard to exploring her life of devotion to others. It takes a long time for her to get in touch with feelings long buried. One memory is a day her family had planned some community rescue mission and she didn't want to go because she was excited about attending a friend's birthday party. Not only did she have to pass on the party, but she got scolded in front of her siblings for being selfish. Over time, more recollections of her protests or those of her siblings come back to her and each one is painful, as she begins to understand that what she has buried is toxic yet has become the foundation for her life.

The inner pressure to do good works has shaped Miriam's life to the point that it has crowded out all other aspects of self. We talk about hobbies and passions and she takes up the cause of finding leisure interests, finally settling on a return to volleyball and a newly identified yearning to travel. The first place she visits is China, on a group tour with friends. Interestingly, she comes back twenty pounds thinner, sleeping like a baby, and announcing that she's made the decision to become a vegan and "have some fun before I die." Not only does she look lighter, but her new more carefree spirit is shining through her.

What's Next? *In Chapter 11, "Finish First, Not Fat,"*
you'll learn

• The attitudes and skills you need to be less nice to others
  and nicer to yourself

- How to handle negative reactions to de-nicing yourself

- How taking better care of yourself will improve your relationship with food and help you maintain a healthy, comfortable weight for life

ELEVEN

Look at Me . . . I'm at the Head of the Line

Finish First, Not Fat

Now that you're almost done with this book, what better time to talk about what you need to do to finish first, not last. You have two major tasks: to cultivate positive self-care attitudes and habits that will keep ratcheting up your self-esteem *and* to break the link between stress and food. Each of these efforts on its own takes a humongous amount of patience and perseverance. To achieve both, you'll have to use all your brainpower, courage, motivation, energy, and single-mindedness. You know, the same qualities you put into being so darned nice and taking such good care of others. How fun—now you get to use them for your own good to maximize your own potential.

Think of all the occasions you've put yourself out for others, barreling right past nice straight into sainthood and martyr-dom. You've proved your capability over and over in the her-culean tasks you've taken on at work and for family, friends, and community. You, of all people, know how to set an agenda and get things done, keep pushing and pushing 'til you reach your goals—for others. Now it's time to use those same top-notch skills to turn the tables on nice and fat and give back to yourself.

You might find it easier to believe that you'll succeed if I break down the abilities you need to finish first. You probably don't realize how many of them you already have and use all the time. And, what you don't have, you'll learn. After all, you didn't get this far in life without being adaptive and resource-ful. So now it's time to use some of that elbow grease on your-self!

▐ GRAB YOUR THINKING CAP How are you feeling in the hope department about chucking your nicey-niceness and learning how to take better care of yourself? What's your take on breaking the link between nice and stress and food? ▐

Can't I just join TDNA—Too Darned Nice Anonymous?

Even if there were such a group (and it's not a bad idea), you'd still have to learn the skills to let go of an identity you've clung to for decades, no easy task. Changing a behavior here or there is a cinch compared to transforming your self-concept, which is the way you see yourself, your identity, what you want to project out into the world about who you are. Some women simply adore being told they're nice, while others want to be thought of as intelligent, creative, savvy, sexy, beautiful, tal-ented, brave, brilliant, well-rounded, altruistic, successful, well-adjusted, a woman for all seasons, or all of the above.

▌ **GRAB YOUR THINKING CAP** What image do you want to project? Are you surprised at how you want to be viewed? How does your image get in the way of finishing first, not fat? ▌

In many ways, the processes of becoming a woman who finishes first and of achieving emotional health are remarkably alike. The main difference is that you have to pay extra special attention to your weakness of wanting to be viewed as nice. That will be your default setting for a very long time (maybe always), but it doesn't mean you can't reprogram yourself every time you slip into good-girl mode. So let's get down to business and see what you need to do to elbow yourself up to the front of the line.

Be self-reflective

Being reflective means keeping an eye on yourself while you're doing what you're doing. It's as if you're holding up a mirror and evaluating your thoughts, feelings, and behaviors even as you're going about everyday life. For example, say your friend calls (for the third time this week) while you've (finally) gotten into doing your taxes, which are due next week, and begs you to babysit for her three-year-old so she can scoot out to get those fabulous Manolo pumps she saw on sale downtown. A reflective person will consider her reaction to such a request before answering. For purposes of reflection, in this example, it doesn't matter whether you say yes or no. What's important is that you're constantly assessing what you think and do and how you feel and don't act automatically.

Reflection is like having a video camera running 24/7 that feeds you info about yourself in real time. Of course, sometimes you might get so caught up in the moment that you can't watch the video and even forget that it's creating footage. Okay, then, when you have a minute, you simply rewind it, review it, and reflect. If you said no to your friend in the above example, you might notice feeling proud but guilty. If you said yes, you might be aware of feeling annoyed at yourself or at her and hopeful that she is appreciative. Most likely, you'll find yourself experiencing a mix of emotions.

Reflecting requires existing on two parallel tracks at once: the doing, thinking, or feeling, and observing these activities. It takes a while to get the hang of it, but after some time, it will feel more natural. The goal is not to become so bogged down in every moment that observation and assessment cut into the flow of your life (Should I put on my right shoe first or my left? Go to the grocery aisle now or the frozen foods?) but to alternate fluidly among acting, feeling, and thinking *and* reflecting on these processes. Without reflection, the door to change remains shut. How can you do things differently if you don't know *what* you're doing? How can you change feelings if you're clueless about what they are? Contemplation gives you the objective feedback you need to notice progress, stuckness, and slippage back to your nice default setting. It's an essential ingredient to the change process.

▌**GRAB YOUR THINKING CAP** How would you rate yourself on reflection? Remember, it's not judging yourself but objectively observing and assessing. ▌

Be compassionate toward yourself

Yes, you've read about compassion before in this book, but I can't bring it up often enough. Nice girls are soooo hard on themselves, so brimming with sympathy and concern for other people (animals, too) and sadly lacking in it toward themselves. If ever there was an imbalance in you, it's in this area. Someone else makes a faux pas and you rush to rescue her from bad feelings, assuring her that everyone makes mistakes and that you don't think less of her for hers. *You*, however, make that same faux pas and you're ready to dunk your head in the toilet or take a galloping leap off a rooftop. Other people are allowed to mess up and fail, but you—never!

You live by two sets of rules: one for you and one for everyone else. The situation wouldn't be so skewed if you weren't so darned over the top nice with others who goof up, perfecting forgiveness and empathy to an art form. So tell me, do you believe that compassion helps other people? If it's good enough for folks you love (or strangers), how come it's not good enough for you? Does it make sense to live with such a double standard?

To finish first it's time to take that same oozing of sympathy and mercy and turn it inward. I can hear your screams across the miles. *Oh, no, let myself off the hook? Yeegads, I couldn't possibly ease off on myself. How could I do as much if I didn't constantly crack the whip over my head? What will people think?* Put your whip away before you get whiplash and, instead, whip out some compassion. You know, as in, I'm doing the best I can, I'm allowed to make mistakes, I tried and failed, I'm going to be okay even though I made a boo-boo. Trust me, self-compassion will serve you far better than self-punishment.

It's ironic that you excel at compassion but forget to use it on yourself. Actually, it's not a matter of not remembering, but not believing you deserve it. Think about it: You're convinced punishment works better for you even though you've been punishing yourself for your transgressions—especially for abusing food and being fat—for decades and you still have food and weight problems.

Give compassion a try. You can always return to flagellating yourself. I promise you won't forget how. But you won't be able to finish first or stop messing yourself up with food until you learn how to be kinder to you. It's just as important as learning to connect to appetite signals such as hunger and fullness. Moreover, once you begin to enjoy being nice to yourself, you won't believe how good it feels and will be horrified (I hope not too horrified) that you've lived so long showering everyone with nice except you.

■ **GRAB YOUR THINKING CAP** Do you tend to be hard on yourself? What do you fear will happen if you give yourself the compassion you give others? ■

Be curious rather than judgmental about your attitudes and behaviors

Along with self-compassion you need a large dollop of self-curiosity. Can you see how reflection, compassion, and curiosity all link together to advance self-understanding and channel your energies toward change? As a nice girl, you generally love to ask people about themselves. I've heard you. You're terrific at problem solving and use your natural inquisitiveness to get answers—for other people. You like to know the internal workings of others so you can help them. What about you?

When you're curious, your mind is wide open to resolution. The reason that curiosity is so useful for nice girls is that you can't be curious and judgmental at the same time! Curiosity opens a window to circulate new ideas, while judgment closes windows, keeps information out, and makes you stagnate. When you've eaten the dessert that you'd been saving for your dinner guests and have to run out at the last minute to buy another, tell me, which is more productive: (a) to obsess about how bad you were and think about hurling yourself under a truck, or (b) to wonder what made you so stressed and uncomfortable that you did something that wasn't in your long-term best interest? Okay, that was a no-brainer, but I hope it shows you how curiosity trumps judgment.

If you want to finish first and become a "normal" eater, you need to understand what attracts you (even unconsciously) to unhealthy eating and finishing last. You have to dig deep, then dig deeper still, until you have all the answers. When you do, your issues will resolve more easily. Being curious about yourself encourages self-reflection, just as ongoing contemplation provides space for you to wonder what makes you tick.

▌ **GRAB YOUR THINKING CAP** Do you tend to be judgmental or curious about yourself? Which has the bigger payoff for attitudinal and behavioral change? ▌

Be self-focused

Notice how much of what you must do involves the word "self"? No accident there. To be self-focused doesn't preclude being other-focused. To be a healthy, balanced person, you must be both. However, all the time you've been taking care of others, you've lost ground focusing on you. I'm not encouraging you to be self-centered or self-absorbed, full of yourself, narcissistic, arrogant, or a Ms. Smarty Pants Know It All whom no one will like (including me). I am saying that you're going to have to start paying lots more attention to your wants and needs.

Again, note how being self-focused implies that you have reflected on your inner workings and have been curious enough to know what your desires are. Being self-focused means getting to know every inch of yourself, understanding yourself as best you can by staying connected to what brings you pleasure and pain and every feeling in between. Focusing on self means facing things such as

- I know I'm supposed to love my father/husband/child/ neighbor, but often I don't.

- I'm exhausted though I haven't done much today.

- I hate salads even though I eat one every day for lunch.

- I'm in a dilemma hating my job but wanting to hold on until retirement.

- I'm terrified of commitment but at the same time I'm awfully lonely.

- I'm not getting any younger and have so many regrets.

- It's time to let go of my old dreams, which will never come true.

- I'm scared of failing, of being disliked, and of so many things in life.

- I'm depressed and have been for decades.

- I had a traumatic childhood that I've never adequately dealt with.

- Most of my friends like me because I do so much for them.

- My life is way out of control.

- I'd love to take risks, but am afraid I'll make mistakes or fail.

- I want a divorce.

- I don't like myself very much.

- I want to change but don't know how.

- My life is a mess.

I didn't say that focusing on yourself would be a picnic. Sometimes it is and sometimes it isn't. The idea is just to keep scanning and handling whatever comes up. If you find something wonderful about yourself, great, go out and celebrate (but not with food!). If you discover something less than endearing, don't ruminate over it and beat yourself up—do something about it. Staying focused means being with yourself in a new way that cannot happen unless you're willing to give up perfection and compromise with being human. Part of the work is identifying authentic feelings, the dreams and desires you've buried under tons of denial and magical thinking, and whatever slim hopes you still have left for a brighter future. Some of what you find will scare the heck out of you, but the rest will make your heart want to go out and do a jig.

▌ **GRAB YOUR THINKING CAP** How often do you stop and focus on your desires and wishes? Does focusing on yourself make you uncomfortable? Why? ▌

Trust yourself

The way we learn to trust ourselves is to trust ourselves. I'm not being a wise guy, I swear. What I mean is that trust builds through experience. You learn from everything you do (or don't do). You did it right, you did it wrong—doesn't matter because whatever happened adds another page to the history of what you know about yourself and how to live. Of course, you have to stay focused on what's going on inside you and reflect on your behavior to get smart and gain self-trust. You can't keep your radar on only sometimes, then turn it off when you feel like it. Like that video camera, it has to keep running 24/7. By staying in touch with your emotions, including your longings, fears, and reactions, you know exactly where you are in situations and relationships. You're like a computer, always integrating new information into programs to keep up to date. Trust comes from being well informed, which means being open to information—whether it comes from within or without—not from burying your head (or heart) in the sand and certainly not from salving your wounds with food.

Mostly trust comes from analyzing actions and consequences. You can't regularly ask other people if you did okay, whether you were right, or how they think things went and expect to develop self-trust. When clients ask me what I think, I often tell them that when I analyze things I build my character, but when they analyze themselves they build theirs. Nice girls are often very, very unsure of themselves. Are you? Being a second-guesser, you ask other people (who usually don't have the psychological savvy to turn the question back to you) what they think, further undermining your own views. And round and round you go until you don't know which end is up.

In order to develop self-trust, you have to take a hiatus from asking people their opinion about things you do and say. Taking a break doesn't mean you can't resume after a while and balance out others' opinions with yours. But you've got to get out there and use your own noodle for a while to teach yourself you're fully capable of deciding for yourself your worth and value, whichever way the coin flips. Sometimes you'll be thrilled to discover that you're a pretty good egg after all; other times, you'll be disappointed that you let yourself down. Either way, the learning is yours and no one can take that away.

▌ **GRAB YOUR THINKING CAP** Do you look to yourself to assess your behavior or turn frequently to others for reassurance? How big an issue is lack of self-trust? How does self-doubt and second-guessing contribute to your being overly nice? ▌

Take risks

This probably comes as no surprise, but nice girls aren't big risk takers. You like to play things safe, you prefer to keep the stuff of life neat and tidy, and you *love* being in control. Often you're attracted to people—friends, lovers, spouses—who are the opposite, who don't worry a lot about consequences or what people think. A part of you would like to be more like them, and the other part simply shudders at the thought of climbing out on some of the limbs they dangle from. Now, I'm not suggesting you rush out and empty your savings account into a Las Vegas slot machine or take up bungee jumping, but I am advising you to loosen up. You may be so worried about consequences and how others will judge you that you're paralyzed when it comes to breaking out of your nice girl role.

To escape this mind-set, you have to start taking teeny, tiny risks. Next time someone is rude to you, don't smile back. You don't need to twist his ears off, but you also don't have to act as if he did you a favor. Refuse to do something you always do—make coffee, do the laundry, take the dog for a walk, clean up your kids' toys, drive your teenagers somewhere at the last minute when you have other plans, stay late at work, give someone a lift when it's way out of your way, plan a get-together, make a cake from scratch, let a whiner complain, scour the house from top to bottom before company comes, buy an expensive gift for someone you don't like. I could go on and on. There are so many things you can refuse to do that will eventually leapfrog you up to the front of the line.

I understand it's scary to take risks. Start small, but also begin thinking about the bigger ones. Maybe you've been un-happy in your marriage for decades. It's okay to think about hurting your spouse's feelings and disappointing your kids and going into counseling or considering leaving. Perhaps you've hated your job or your profession and have given up hope of ever finding a satisfying career. Just start noodling around in your head what you *might* do for a living. Could be you've been wanting to move to another part of the country. You don't need to plan a yard sale yet. Instead, daydream about where you might want to live. Get the picture? Take the risk in your head where there aren't any consequences until you're ready to move into real-world action.

▌ **GRAB YOUR THINKING CAP** Are you scared of taking risks because you might make a mistake, fail, be wrong? How does that keep you a nice girl? ▌

Find balance

Life is never perfectly in balance. Well, maybe for a nanosecond, but not much longer. Something always comes up to throw us off course, but that's okay. Because life isn't static, our job is to keep adjusting as it moves us along. When it moves us to the right, we need to compensate and come back a little to the left, and vice versa. The idea is not to stay rigidly in the middle or at either extreme for long. In fact, a healthy life is much like a pendulum. Give it a hard push and it makes a full, wide swing from one end of its arc to another. Give it a gentle shove and it passes back and forth over the center in smaller arcs.

Think of regulating yourself as if you were a pendulum. One day you're a slug and never get out of bed, reading mys-tery after mystery, while the next day you're out from dawn 'til dusk and feel pleasantly exhausted when you hit the sack. If you don't like going to extremes, keep your arc shorter by balancing each day with uptime and downtime. Let yourself rest in the center, then give yourself a nudge in one direction, say, having dinner out with friends twice in a week, then moving in the other direction by staying in two nights in a row.

Balance doesn't have to occur every day or even every week. Some periods are naturally busier than others. But you want to experience harmony with yourself and your environment from the inside out. You want to aim for a sense of satisfaction and equilibrium that comes from regulating your life between time spent with and doing for others and time set aside for being with and doing for yourself. You'll have to remain self-focused and reflective to find the nuances of balance. You'll have to encourage yourself to take risks and be compassionate with yourself when you under- and overdo. Ain't it grand how learning one skill gives you a chance to work on all the others?

▌GRAB YOUR THINKING CAP How good are you at keeping your life in balance? What throws you off? What do you need to do to stay on a more even keel? ▌▌

Be emotionally uncomfortable

Paradoxically, the hardest part of change is exactly what you need to do for it to happen: experience uncomfortable feelings. If you're not willing to do that (or at least give it the old college try), you might as well set this book aside. My suggestion is to think about your ability to tolerate painful emotions and then either work on improving it on your own or find a therapist to help you. If you've had trauma in your life, I would definitely go the therapist route. If you haven't experienced trauma, you might be able to keep stretching yourself gradually to tolerate more and more intense discomfort.

In order to change we need awareness and discomfort. Unfortunately, when feelings get too strong, we generally tune out, often with food. As you can see, not eating emotionally will provide opportunities for you to feel your feelings, so long as you don't rush off to silence them some other way. To be an emotionally healthy person, which includes knowing when to play the nice card and when not to, you need to stay in touch with feelings. This is not optional work. It is a must. It will not happen overnight, but it is definitely doable over time with reflection, self-focus, curiosity, and self-compassion. Through having confidence in your ability to know yourself, you'll develop self-trust and get in better balance. It all fits together so, well, nicely, doesn't it?

■ **GRAB YOUR THINKING CAP** How well do you experience distressing or painful emotions? How does this ability (or inability) relate to being overnice and to your eating and weight problems? ■

If I'm less nice, does that mean there will be less of me to be nice?

If you're asking if I'm offering you some sort of weight-loss plan, the answer is a resounding no. Overweight is a lot more complicated than simply resigning from half your volunteer activities and telling your husband to pick up his underwear. Weight is a complex issue that is a combination of genetics, lifestyle, socialization, metabolism, habit, and nutrition. However, I'll go so far as to say that by being *automatically* less nice, you'll be taking better care of yourself, which will reduce your stress and tendency to de-stress through eating. All other factors being equal, it makes sense that by decreasing mindless eating, you'll lose weight, but I can't guarantee it.

You have two major tasks ahead of you: (1) not stressing yourself out so much by being nice, and (2) not turning to food when you are stressed. You'll have to develop other strategies to cope with feeling upset, overwhelmed, disappointed, con-flicted, hurt, and anxious if you plan to put food in its proper place, which is for fuel and pleasure. If you're serious about taking off weight—and, more important, keeping it off—you'll need a repertoire of tried-and-true techniques and habits that will help you regulate emotions and respond effectively to life's ups and downs. Without them, even if you manage to keep your niceness down to an acceptable level, you'll still return to food-seeking behavior when you hit a bump in the road.

Developing self-care strategies is not a one-size-fits all matter. Mostly it's trial and error and figuring out what works for you. I love to read, but occasionally when I'm antsy, TV lulls me into la-la land better than any book ever could. I exercise regularly, but it's not an activity I'd seek out when I'm upset. Generally, I work through problems by experiencing my feel-ings to the max and talking them over with people I trust. And when I'm stuck and can't seem to make my life work the way I want it to, I don't hesitate to return to therapy. Now, these are *my* strategies and they work for *me* (most of the time), but they won't necessarily work for you.

A good way to figure out what kind of self-care you need is to think in terms of whether you want to be alone or with people. Sometimes a quick cup of coffee and a schmooze with a friend is just the thing. Other times it will take you away from whatever emotions you're trying to connect with. Another method is to decide whether you need to calm down because you're careening around like a pinball or could use an energy boost because you're sinking into apathy and the blues. Self-care would be very different in each instance. You can't just pick one strategy out of the air and expect it to succeed all the time. It has to match your need and your mood. If you need to cry, watching a comedy on TV will only postpone the inevitable; however, if you've been bawling for days, a good laugh might jolt you out of the doldrums.

By making eating the *last* activity you turn to when you're stressed or upset, you have a good shot at improving your relationship with food. Sure, everyone eats once in a while for emotional reasons, so please cut yourself some slack. But you want to create enough pathways out of distress that you don't make a beeline to the fridge every time life throws you a curve ball. Effective self-care will happen only when you have a plan that includes effective options and then follow it diligently.

As I said, improving self-care is one of the major tasks ahead of you. The other is not turning to food when you're stressed or going through any kind of emotional discomfort. By improving self-care techniques, you'll reduce stress some, but you still have to work on resolving your eating problems if you want to lead a happy, healthy life. My first suggestion is to stop dieting and obsessing about weight and, instead, throw your energy into learning to eat "normally." I recommend my book *The Rules of "Normal" Eating: A Commonsense Approach for Dieters, Overeaters, Undereaters, Emotional Eaters, and Everyone in Between!* which is full of excellent information about nearly every aspect of your relationship with food and your body.

In a nutshell, along with learning to manage your feelings without food, you'll need to learn to eat only when you're hungry, choose satisfying foods, eat with awareness and enjoyment, and stop when you're full or satisfied. This may seem like a tall order for someone with a lifetime of food struggles. Dieting isn't the long-term answer. The majority of people who diet to lose weight regain it, often putting back on more pounds than they originally lost. Moreover, dieting sets up your body for conserving calories and rebound eating. The only way out of the diet-binge cycle is to teach your appetite to regulate your food intake. This process is learnable over a period of many months to a few years. It's not a quick fix, but it definitely does work. The nondiet approach to weight loss has been around since the late 1970s and is a slow but steady process that moves you toward achieving and maintaining a comfortable, healthy weight for life.

I learned to become a "normal" eater myself many decades ago and have practiced it ever since. I don't do it perfectly but am proud to say that I'm no longer an emotional eater. My weight is stable and I don't obsess about food, but the best bonus is that my emotions are now available to steer me toward health and happiness.

▮ **GRAB YOUR THINKING CAP** What are your eating goals? (Notice I didn't ask about your weight goals!) What have you done to meet them? What are you willing to do to become a "normal" eater? ▮

Are people going to like me finishing first or being at the head of the line?

I understand your question, but it's still part of nice girl–think. It's not a matter of people liking you, but of *you* liking you. The rule of thumb is that true intimates and people who want the best for you will be tickled pink that you've finally taken your rightful place in the world. They've been hoping you'd see the light and pushing you to take better care of yourself all along. As to other people, well, some will be in shock and won't know what to make of your newfound confidence, assertion, and pride. When they come out of shock, they will hopefully realize that your changes are for the best—for you and for them. Other people are so focused on themselves that they won't even notice you're different. Really, there are people out there, unlike you, who don't pay much attention to what other people do or think, don't make judgments, and are happier in their own world than peering into yours.

Then there are the folks whose lives will shift dramatically because you're coming into your own and standing up for yourself. Many of them will be unhappy, scared, or enraged that you've found your voice and your stride. Some will tell you exactly what they think about your selfishness (over and over and over). They'll sulk and act disappointed, play the victim to try and suck you back into taking care of them, puff up and get all entitled and even more demanding, and try their very best to cut you down to size.

Need I admonish that these are not people who have your interest at heart? If you can, reduce the amount of time you're with them or stay away from them completely (for now). Gradually, some of these folks will grudgingly come around and accept the new you. However, some never will. Do your duty but no more with them; I don't care how they're associated with or related to you. If you have to be around them, be aware beforehand that they're going to test your limits and be prepared to hold your ground. Rehearse what you're going to say to them and do something supernice for yourself after you've done your duty. Think of it as combat pay!

■ **GRAB YOUR THINKING CAP** Make a list of your allies in finishing first, folks who won't care much or even notice, and people who're going to fight you tooth and nail. What are you going to do to get reinforcement from your allies, win over and make cheerleaders of people who may not care a lot, and depower your foes? ■

I hope you're as excited for yourself as I am for you. Sure you're scared and maybe a bit overwhelmed. You have no idea if you're going to be able to make the changes you want to and there's no certainty that you're going to succeed. But think what will happen when you do! You'll be a more well-rounded person, your stress level will plummet, you'll have more time for yourself and your passions, you'll feel happier, lighter, more satisfied, and prouder of who you are. Plus, your chances of slimming down and staying there will be better than ever. Not bad for giving up nice, huh?

Aren't you going to give me a No More Nice Girl Manifesto for finishing first?

No. I've done my job by teaching you the ways being a nice girl contributes to putting others' needs before your own and how to de-nice and take better care of yourself. You now have the basics for taking your show on the road, so it's your turn to write your own manifesto. Think of it. Your manifesto will be like no other because it will be tailored to you—to your specific excesses of goodness, your gifts and talents, and your uniqueness and specialness.

Good luck! See you up there at the front of the line!

To do today

Go out and do something positively special for yourself that makes you feel a little bit naughty.

NO MORE NICE GIRL MANIFESTO FOR _____ (NAME)

DO

- _____
- _____
- _____
- _____
- _____
- _____
- _____
- _____
- _____

DON'T

- _____
- _____
- _____

- _____

- _____

- _____

- _____

- _____

- _____

- _____

Meet One of the Nice Girls

Samantha now

At seventy-one, Samantha came to therapy as what she calls "my last resort." Married to a man she often likes, but never loved, she finds that the older she gets, the angrier she feels but she can't figure out why. She describes her life as neither terribly bad nor very good. Having spent most of it trying to do the right thing, she can't understand what she's so furious about, describing herself as walking around "half the time wanting to bite someone's head off." When we talk about her marital dissatisfactions and I lightly mention the possibility of "divorce," she gives me an adamant, "No!" Although she agrees that her marriage is far from perfect, she maintains that, in fact, her life with her husband is somewhat better now that they're retired and are less stressed.

Samantha trained as an engineer but stayed home to raise

her son. She wishes she'd continued working in her field but recognizes that it wasn't typical of the times; plus her husband strongly preferred that she focus on being a wife and mother. When her son was grown, she considered trying to teach engineering at a local college, but the educational and credentialing hoops she had to jump through were daunting. Instead she took a job as an assistant to a contractor and felt relatively satisfied.

Though she devoted her time to rearing her son, she's not particularly close with him and wishes he and his family were nearby so she could get to know her three grandchildren. Due to her husband's fear of flying, the two do little in the way of travel and generally see her son's family only when they come for an annual visit. She's asked her son to visit more often, but he owns a business and says he can't get away. She doesn't feel at ease enough with her daughter-in-law to call and invite her to visit with her children without him.

Samantha is remarkably in touch with her emotions, at least with her anger, if not the more vulnerable sentiments beneath it. She describes gobbling down platefuls of food and loving to chomp away at foods that are hard and crispy. Recently, she broke a tooth when she crunched down on an overtoasted bagel. Because she's been slim most of her life, she's uncomfortable with having gained ten pounds in the last year, both for health reasons and because her clothes no longer fit. When she mentions her discomfort to her husband, he shrugs and says she's fine the way she is.

Samantha as a child

She grew up in a dysfunctional family. Her mother was highly narcissistic and ignored her daughter except to criticize her. Instead, her mother devoted herself to Samantha's exceptionally gifted brother who entered college when he was twelve.

Nothing was too good for him and Samantha grew up in his considerable shadow. Although she had a loving relationship with her father, he was at work most of the time and she never saw enough of him. She was fond of her brother but also resented the attention he received from her mother and from the rest of the world.

Neither assertive nor competitive by nature, she did what she was told and accepted her lot in life. It was through her father's encouragement that she became an engineer, and she considers her degree her crowning achievement (she is prouder of it than of her son). She was nearly thirty when her husband came along and when he asked to marry her, she accepted. "That's what young women did back then," she tells me with a sigh, "you know, before women's lib." When it seemed the right time, she got pregnant and had a child.

De-nicing Samantha

Although this is her first time in therapy, Samantha works as if she's making up for lost time, which she is. She's eager to learn all about herself when she realizes that much of her is buried deep below the surface. When I lift the lid off her anger, we find resentment, sadness, disappointment, regrets, and more regrets. Samantha realizes she's been seething for decades but has kept her rage under wraps. We finally stumble upon what freed her anger: the wedding of a friend's daughter. The daughter had coincidentally also trained as an engineer and had taken a job at a notable firm with the blessings of her husband. Somehow, Samantha recalls, "That did it. She was making the choices I wish I'd made. I remember eating my dessert that night and grabbing my husband's and eating that, too. I think that was my first rebellious act."

Samantha asked her husband to join us for a therapy session, but he refused, saying she had to settle her problems on her own. She was disappointed and told him so. She also called her son and said she wanted to get to know her grandchildren before they grew up. Although he promised to bring the children for a visit, he's been slow to firm up plans, but Samantha intends to stay on him until he does. When she didn't get what she wanted from him, she contacted her daughter-in-law and they've established a lovely, intimate relationship that has warmed Samantha's heart and brings tears to her eyes when she talks about it.

The biggest change is that her anger has subsided. She's lost the weight she gained and is back to eating "normally." She knows it's too late to have the life she wanted, but she is willing to work to have the best life she can have for whatever time she has left. She thinks it's funny that I've written a book called *Nice Girls Finish Fat* and kids me that the book is all about her.

References

1. Kolata, Gina. *Rethinking Thin: The New Science of Weight Loss—and the Myths and Realities of Dieting.* (New York: Farrar, Straus, & Giroux, 2007).
2. National Organization for Women, *Women Deserve Equal Pay*, retrieved 4/22/08, www.now.org.
3. Brownmiller, Susan. *Femininity.* (New York: Ballantine Books, 1984).

Index

About the Author

Karen R. Koenig, LCSW, M.Ed., is a cognitive-behavioral therapist, eating coach, educator, author, and speaker—an expert on
the psychology of eating—with thirty years' experience teaching chronic dieters and emotional eaters the skills that "normal"
eaters use naturally to maintain a comfortable, healthy weight
for life.

Koenig is the author of *The Rules of "Normal" Eating: A
Commonsense Approach for Dieters, Overeaters, Undereaters, Emotional
Eaters, and Everyone in Between!*, *The Food and Feelings Workbook:
A Full Course Meal on Emotional Health*, and *What Every Therapist
Needs to Know About Treating Eating and Weight Issues*. Her articles
and essays have appeared in *Social Work Focus*, *Social Work Today*,
Eating Disorders Today, the *Society for Family Therapy and Research*
newsletter, the *Boston Globe*, the *Boston Herald*, *Attitudes* maga-
zine, and *Positive Change*. A founding member of the Greater
Boston Collaborative for Body Image and Eating Disorders, she
served on the Professional Advisory Board of the multiservice
Eating Disorder Association of Massachusetts.

For three decades, Ms. Koenig has been teaching eating
workshops for the general public and has lectured at Simmons
College School of Social Work, Boston University School
of Social Work, the Massachusetts School of Professional
Psychology, the National Association of Social Work, the
Massachusetts Dietetic Association, the National Organization
for Women, the Massachusetts Eating Disorder Association,
and the University of South Florida Social Work Department.

A graduate of Simmons College School of Social Work,

Ms. Koenig practices and teaches in Sarasota, Florida. Learn more about her at www.eatingnormal.com, www.nicegirls finishfat.com, and www.squidoo.com/eatnormalnow. Read her blogs at www.eatingdisordersblogs.com and join her message board at http://groups.yahoo.com/group/foodand feelings.